The Handbook (

Eating, Drinking
and Swallowing Problems
in Adults with Fibromyalgia

© 2023 J&R Press Ltd

British Library Cataloguing in Publication Data
A catalogue record for this book is available from the British Library
Book and cover design: Jim Wilkie.
(Cover image used under license from Shutterstock.com)

Index compiled by Terence Halliday
hallidayterence@aol.com

Printed and bound by CPI Group (UK) Ltd, Croydon, CR0 4YY

The Handbook of
Eating, Drinking and Swallowing Problems in Adults with Fibromyalgia

Órla Gilheaney

and

Kathleen Mc Tiernan

J&R Press Ltd

Contents

5 How can healthcare professionals support people with fibromyalgia-associated dysphagia?

Órla Gilheaney, Ellen Carroll and Kathleen Mc Tiernan

6 The future of collaborative care provision and research into fibromyalgia-associated dysphagia _____ 43

Órla Gilheaney and Kathleen Mc Tiernan

Acknowledgements

Firstly, we wish to thank all of the people who took part in the studies referenced in this book. In addition, we would like to extend our thanks to the people who participated in and helped to organise the FibroForum in Trinity College Dublin in May 2022. Many thanks also to our co-authors of chapters. Finally, we would like to extend our sincere thanks to J&R Press for supporting us in writing this book.

1 Eating, drinking, and swallowing problems experienced by people living with fibromyalgia

Kathleen Mc Tiernan and Órla Gilheaney

1.1 How are fibromyalgia and swallowing linked?

Fibromyalgia and swallowing difficulties are two concepts which are rarely discussed simultaneously; however, for many people living with fibromyalgia, swallowing problems are a daily challenge that often goes unmentioned and untreated. For some people living with fibromyalgia, even the most simple pleasure of sharing a cup of tea or coffee and a chat with a friend becomes a stressful, difficult and, in some cases, even dangerous activity. Despite the potential for serious outcomes, swallowing difficulties in this group are rarely discussed between patients and their healthcare providers, treated explicitly, or adequately researched. Because of this lack of research and reporting, there is limited awareness of the potential for the development of fibromyalgia-associated swallowing difficulties. This handbook on fibromyalgia and swallowing problems compiles recent research and patient-lived experience, and suggests some coping strategies for people with fibromyalgia-associated swallowing problems, their carers, and clinicians. The aim of this book is to inform, empower, and inspire people living with, caring for, or treating someone with swallowing problems associated with fibromyalgia, with the ultimate goal of improving quality of life, health outcomes, and participation in activities of daily living.

1.2 What is fibromyalgia?

Fibromyalgia is a chronic disease that causes pain, fatigue, and tenderness all over the body. It is the second most prevalent 'rheumatic' disorder after osteoarthritis (Clauw, 2014), and it is common for fibromyalgia to co-occur with other rheumatic conditions like lupus, osteoarthritis and rheumatoid arthritis, with between 10-30% of people with these rheumatic disorders also meeting the conditions for a diagnosis of fibromyalgia (Clauw, 2014). Although co-occurrence of fibromyalgia with other diseases is common, it also often presents as the primary condition, independent of any other diagnoses. Fibromyalgia is extremely common; its reported prevalence is 2-8% of the population. People with fibromyalgia have histories of chronic pain throughout their bodies that typically began in adolescence or young adulthood (Bhargava & Hurley, 2022).

Pain is the most common symptom of fibromyalgia; however, people with fibromyalgia often experience difficulties with cognitive functioning, sleep disruption, mood alterations, and sensitivity to external stimuli (Sarzi-Puttini, Giorgi, Marotto, & Atzeni, 2020). People with fibromyalgia can also have other significant health challenges, such as temporomandibular disorders, migraine, and irritable bowel syndrome (Häuser et al., 2015). In addition to these challenging physical symptoms, fibromyalgia can also have a negative influence on psychological wellbeing, the ability to create and sustain meaningful relationships and quality of life (Galvez-Sánchez, Duschek, & Reyes Del Paso, 2019). The severity of the disorder varies from one individual to the next depending on the combination of symptoms a person is experiencing and the extent of the impact that the combination of symptoms has on their daily lives.

Fibromyalgia is often classed as a 'rheumatic' disease due to its symptomatic similarity to conditions such as rheumatoid arthritis (e.g., pain, reduced mobility, fatigue). However, evidence has now shown that fibromyalgia is in fact not a condition of widespread inflammation or simply a psychological manifestation of trauma, but an issue with the 'final common pathway', or sensitization of the nervous system, resulting in amplified pain signals being sent from the brain to the peripheral parts of the body in the absence of ongoing peripheral input. This results in chronic pain, and associated issues, due to amplified brain signals despite there being no ongoing 'injury' (Tracey & Bushnell, 2009; Woolf, 2011). Fibromyalgia is diagnosed by assessing patient history and by physical examination (Arout, Sofuoglu, Bastian, & Rosenheck, 2018). Traditionally, the key diagnostic indicator is the experience of pain, when palpated, in at least 11 of the 18 tender points around the body, which has persisted for at least three months (Rhodus, Fricton, Carlson, & Messner, 2003). In addition to the palpation assessment, severity rating scales, which are based on the American College of Rheumatology (ARC) diagnostic criteria, are used to assess the extent and impact of the disease state. Fibromyalgia affects six times as many females as it does males and it can occur at any age. Its prevalence is similar across countries and ethnicities. People who have close relatives with fibromyalgia are eight times more likely to have fibromyalgia or chronic pain, therefore genetic (inherited) factors may increase the likelihood of having fibromyalgia at some point across the lifespan.

1.3 What is dysphagia?

Normal swallowing typically happens across four phases: (1) the oral preparatory phase (where the food/drink is taken into the mouth); (2) the oral phase (where the food/drink is prepared for swallowing either by chewing and mashing or by scooping fluid together in a way that is easy to swallow); (3) the pharyngeal phase (where the food and drink passes through the throat, towards the food pipe while avoiding the air/windpipe); and (4) the oesophageal phase (where food passes into the food pipe and down into the stomach) (Lancaster, 2015; Sasegbon & Hamdy, 2017; Tomik et al., 2020). Normal swallowing is essential for maintaining optimal nutrition, hydration, and body weight/composition.

Dysphagia is the medical term for 'difficulty swallowing'. It can develop as a result of a number of acquired or idiopathic health conditions, at any stage in life (Sasegbon & Hamdy, 2017). For example, dysphagia can develop secondary to stroke, Parkinson's disease, cerebral palsy, acquired brain injury, head or neck cancer, motor neurone disease, etc. Figures on how common dysphagia is vary due to different patient groups studied, different types of studies carried out, and different ways of reporting findings. It is estimated that dysphagia is experienced by between 2-20% of the general global population (Adkins et al., 2020).

Dysphagia can cause adverse health outcomes, such as malnutrition or dehydration from not eating or drinking enough or aspiration pneumonia from food and/or drink going into the air pipe as opposed to the food pipe (among other issues) (Garand et al., 2020). In addition, dysphagia can also cause significant psychological and emotional issues as many social gatherings centre around meeting for food or drinks, an experience that can be isolating or stressful for people living with dysphagia (Ekberg et al., 2002).

1.4 What is fibromyalgia-associated dysphagia?

Dysphagia and fibromyalgia have rarely been discussed together in the medical literature. In addition, swallowing difficulties have never been included as a symptom that has to be present in order to be able to diagnose someone with fibromyalgia (Arnold et al., 2019; Wolfe et al., 2010). Despite the lack of large-scale research, there have been numerous anecdotal reports and small studies that speak about real-life experiences of fibromyalgia-associated swallowing problems. These accounts discuss how people with fibromyalgia often live with a wide variety of symptoms, such as dry mouth, tongue burning, food and drink tasting unusual/unpleasant, pain on swallowing, sensations of choking, and reflux (Bhadra & Petersel, 2010; Colón León & Centeno Vázquez, 2021; Jalilvand, Belle, McNally, & Perry, 2019; Piersala, Akst, Hillel, & Best, 2020; Rhodus, Fricton, Carlson, & Messner, 2003; Seccia, Rossitto, Calò, & Rossi, 2015). This wide variety of experiences suggests that patients may be living with a myriad of issues that could impact not only on eating and drinking but also on psychosocial wellbeing and participation in normal social, personal, or work-related occasions.

Research has not yet fully clarified why people with fibromyalgia may experience swallowing problems. So far, only tentative suggestions about the potential cause of swallowing problems in people with fibromyalgia have been offered. For example, some authors have spoken about the possibility that taking multiple medications may cause unintended swallowing problems, reduced muscular function, and dry mouth (Balasubramaniam, Laudenbach, & Stoopler, 2007). Additionally, it has been suggested that people with fibromyalgia may have increased nervous system sensitivity in their mouth and face that may make it uncomfortable or painful to eat and drink normally (Fitzgerald & Triadafilopoulos, 1997; Vivino et al., 2019), while other authors have spoken about the high prevalence of jaw joint problems among those with fibromyalgia which can make it difficult to chew properly (Jeon, 2020; Sasegbon & Hamdy, 2017). However, despite many competing ideas, there has been no conclusive statement on the definitive cause of these fibromyalgia-related swallowing problems. In addition, although it is positive that studies exist that talk about symptoms and their potential causes, problems have been identified with how these studies were carried out. For example, some studies included only a few participants, which makes it difficult to prove causation and to generalise results to bigger groups. Speech and language therapists were rarely included in the study design or conduct, and the tools they used in assessment of swallowing problems were often not valid or reliable (Gilheaney & Chadwick, 2023). Therefore, while it is important to be aware of these studies and to use them as a foundation for future work, we also have to be conscious of their limitations and how these may not tell the full story of living with fibromyalgia-associated swallowing problems. As such, it is more important than ever to go directly to the people with expert knowledge in this area – the people who are living with dysphagia and fibromyalgia. It is essential that the voices of these people are amplified so that we can truly understand their experiences and priorities. With this vital information, patients, researchers, and clinicians can collaborate to plan how to best deliver effective treatment and patient support into the future.

1.5 What are the implications of fibromyalgia-associated dysphagia?

This chapter discussed fibromyalgia, dysphagia, and the potential for how these two conditions can be interlinked. Building on this foundation, the physiological and psychosocial implications of fibromyalgia-associated swallowing problems will be explored in the coming chapters, drawing on patients' real-life accounts, research data, and views from frontline clinicians.

2 Physical signs and symptoms of fibromyalgia-associated dysphagia

Órla Gilheaney, Catherine Costello
and Kathleen Mc Tiernan

2.1 Fibromyalgia-associated swallowing problems: A myriad of complex signs and symptoms

People with fibromyalgia often experience difficulties with eating, drinking, and swallowing. Due to the many different symptoms that people with fibromyalgia live with, it can be hard to know if swallowing difficulties are associated with their chronic pain and fatigue problems. This may lead to a lack of reporting of these issues to their healthcare providers. In addition, due to a lack of research into these issues, healthcare providers may not be aware that many people with fibromyalgia have swallowing problems, leaving them unsure of how to treat these issues or support their patients. To promote awareness of these issues and help to improve reporting and treatment, we outline here the physiological signs and symptoms of fibromyalgia-associated swallowing issues, bringing together previous evidence, recent research, and the patient voice.

2.2 What do we know about fibromyalgia-associated eating and drinking problems?

Until recent years there had been very few research studies carried out that investigated eating, drinking, and swallowing problems among people living with fibromyalgia. This means that there wasn't much objective data available to help us to understand how common these issues are and how they affect the people living with them. In a recent systematic review where all globally available research and reports on this topic were reviewed together and compared (Gilheaney & Chadwick, 2023), researchers found only six relevant studies that had looked at this topic. Typically, in projects like this, the results of all identified studies would be combined in a process known as meta-analysis in order to create a more comprehensive description of the health condition. However, the studies identified here were very varied in how they were carried out, what types of participants they recruited, and their relative quality. This meant that in many cases results could not be compared or combined in this way.

Meta-analysis could only be completed for two out of a total of 12 symptoms studied. Difficulties swallowing were found in 52% of participants, while reflux was present in 26% (Gilheaney & Chadwick, 2023). Interestingly, no studies were identified in this project that discussed patients' experiences of aspiration/penetration (or food and drink going 'the wrong way'), unintentional weight loss, or impaired, painful, or tiring chewing, despite these being commonly reported by patients anecdotally. For other symptoms (e.g., altered taste, tongue burning, painful swallowing, or dry mouth), only one or two studies had been published on these issues or studies recruited too few participants to produce conclusive evidence on how common these issues were.

However, although there wasn't much objective data out there to describe these issues, this did not mean that the issues did not exist. In the absence of available numbers and figures, it was more important than ever for researchers and clinicians to listen to the voices of patients and to seek their views and experiences. As such, recent research on fibromyalgia-associated swallowing problems has been conducted which drew on the expertise of those living with these issues, as discussed in the sections below.

2.3 Recent research on fibromyalgia-associated swallowing problems

An anonymous online survey was carried out in 2021 (Gilheaney, Costello, & Mc Tiernan [In Press]) and 1983 people who were over the age of 18 and living with fibromyalgia participated. People were recruited from fibromyalgia support groups in six different countries (Ireland, the United Kingdom, Australia, New Zealand, Canada, and the United States of America). Participants were asked about their age, gender, location, and their experience of eating, drinking, and swallowing problems. Participants were aged between 18 and 94 years of age, with 95% identifying as female (Figure 2.1).

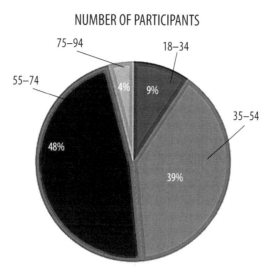

Figure 2.1 Demographics of participants in Gilheaney, Costello, & Mc Tiernan [In Press].

Data was analysed to identify any trends and common experiences of swallowing problems among people with fibromyalgia.

The physical symptoms that participants reported varied, as shown in Figure 2.2.

Regardless of age, all people with fibromyalgia reported experiencing severe eating, drinking, and swallowing problems. The most common experience overall was dry mouth, which can make it difficult to chew and swallow

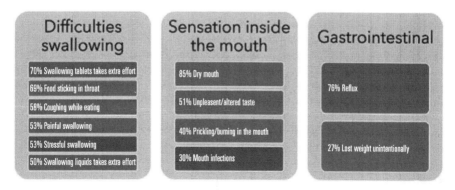

Figure 2.2 Results of Gilheaney, Costello, & Mc Tiernan, [In Press].

food, moisten the mouth, and taste food and drink normally (Gilheaney et al., 2022). These findings were corroborated by a recent qualitative study in which people living with fibromyalgia-associated swallowing problems discussed similar physical symptoms (Hussey & Gilheaney, 2022). Examples of their experience include:

> "The tongue and the whole area gets very dry."

> "At night, I'd probably wake up about eight times a night and have to drink a glass of water because my mouth is so dry."

Generalised swallowing difficulties were often reported in the study by Gilheaney and colleagues (Gilheaney et al., 2022), with the overall difficulties in getting food from one's mouth to their stomach smoothly. Example included issues with swallowing tablets, experiences of food sticking in the throat which may or may not cause pain and can be associated with the need to cough to clear one's throat. Again, this statistical data was backed up by the first-person experiences collected as part of Hussey's (2022) study. Here, real-life accounts from people living with fibromyalgia-associated dysphagia (Hussey & Gilheaney, 2022) brought the data from Costello et al. survey (2022) to life, and told the story of the true difficulties patients experience in living with these issues. For example:

> "And the oval paracetamol capsule's about the biggest I can take, anything bigger than that I would have to break up because it's it I just can't do it. I would be coughing it back out."

> "When I go somewhere, I always explained to people look don't worry, I will cough and I might choke a bit, but it's part of my condition and I can't help it. I try not to, but you know, I'm sorry if I do and it upsets you or embarrasses you or whatever."

> "I get that pain, that little knife pain in the back of my throat."

This study suggested that these symptoms resulted in people with fibromyalgia often experiencing additional worry while eating.

> "But it does worry me because if I choke when I'm on own, and I do stop breathing, or I inhale the drink rather than swallow the drink." (Hussey & Gilheaney, 2022)

These physical and sensory issues can lead to people eating less or eating less nutritionally balanced but soft food (e.g., ice cream, milkshakes, or puddings) and therefore experiencing unintended changes in their body weight, as documented in Costello et al. (2022). Going beyond statistical data, analysis of online comments posted about this topic on patient-led forums suggests that this is a widespread issue, with many people relying on self-modifying their diets so as to continue oral feeding (Gavigan & Gilheaney, 2022). For example:

> "Thank goodness for protein shakes."

> "The blender would also be handy for making food shakes so there are no chunks to scrape on the way down." (Gavigan & Gilheaney, 2022)

These dietary and weight changes can have a knock-on negative effect on other parts of life, for example energy levels, mobility, engaging in physical activity, sleep quality, self-esteem:

> "Oh god yeah, so it just knocks your confidence a bit."

2.4 Synthesising the physical signs and symptoms of fibromyalgia-associated dysphagia

In conclusion, we have outlined here the common signs and symptoms of fibromyalgia-associated swallowing problems. It is clear that these issues are frequently experienced, even if they are not always reported or clinically treated. By pulling together the evidence to date, with consideration of the patient's voice, a spotlight is placed on a common occurrence that is often overlooked by patients and healthcare providers, who focus primarily on issues with weight bearing joints. In the next chapter, we will expand on this discussion to provide an insight to the reality of living with these problems on a daily basis, with consideration of the social, psychological, emotional, functional, and occupational difficulties that come with fibromyalgia-associated swallowing issues.

3 Exploring the lived experience of fibromyalgia and eating, drinking, and swallowing problems

Kathleen Mc Tiernan, Joeann Hussey, Rhianne Gavigan and Órla Gilheaney

3.1 Exploring the research and first-hand patient accounts of the impact of living with chronic illness

This chapter expands on the previous discussion of the common eating, drinking, and swallowing problems experienced by people with fibromyalgia, by exploring previous research and first-hand patient accounts about the psychosocial lived experience of these issues. These real-life patient accounts can help deepen our understanding of the impact of these problems on people's daily lives.

3.2 The lived experiences of chronic illness

Invisible illnesses, especially those which can affect energy and pain levels, are known to impact on people's quality of life and to cause them to have negative lived experiences (Megari, 2013). With regard specifically to fibromyalgia, the experience of a combination of the multiple symptoms associated with this condition can have a negative impact on a person's quality of life and their ability to create sustainable and meaningful relationships (Galvez-Sánchez et al., 2019). The combined multiple symptoms of fibromyalgia can create a substantial invisible obstacle and very often make normal daily living more challenging. There are a number of aspects of daily life that can be impacted by the challenges associated with symptoms of fibromyalgia. Things that most people take for granted are much more difficult for people with chronic illnesses (Diviney & Dowling, 2015).

Independent of fibromyalgia, there is also a significant psychological and social burden caused by dysphagia (Ekberg et al., 2002). People with swallowing problems often have a lower quality of life as a result of the avoidance of communal eating opportunities and the loss of social interaction that communal eating provides (Luca, Smith, & Hibbert, 2022). People who have dysphagia, as a symptom of other neurological issues such as motor neurone disease or Parkinson's disease for example, can have altered perceptions of food that result in negative emotions being associated with the experience of eating (Ninfa et al., 2021). Eating is very often a social experience that is a time for friends and family to gather and share stories about their lives, to share common experiences and to bond. When the physical act of eating and drinking is an uncomfortable and sometimes frightening experience due to a sensation of pain or choking, the social aspects of eating are diminished as the focus shifts to the mechanics of eating a meal. This can lead to people with swallowing problems avoiding social meals, and the fallout of this avoidance is the loss of meaningful social interactions, the pleasures of shared mealtimes, the depth of strong social relationships, and the feelings of wellbeing and overall quality of life.

Studies not specific to fibromyalgia have reported that people prefer to manage the symptoms of swallowing difficulties independently, even though the outcomes for people with dysphagia are much better if they are supported by healthcare specialists (Lisiecka, Kelly, & Jackson, 2021). As people living with fibromyalgia-associated dysphagia have these swallowing problems as only one small part of their overall symptom profile they may not report their swallowing problems to healthcare providers. These people may have to report more overt or pressing issues (e.g., mobility concerns or uncontrolled pain and fatigue) which may lead to swallowing problems not being appropriately treated or managed by the clinician. In turn, this may lead to independent ad hoc compensation for swallowing difficulties and ultimately result in poorer patient outcomes and quality of life as they are not seeking or receiving the expert care that they require. Therefore, it is critically important to amplify people's lived experiences to identify why they prefer to try to deal with their swallowing problems by themselves, especially as research shows that people with dysphagia have better long-term health outcomes if their swallowing problem is treated by healthcare professionals who specialise in this area.

3.3 The lived experiences of fibromyalgia-associated dysphagia

People with fibromyalgia experience poorer health-related quality of life that can be associated with worse psychosocial and overall health outcomes (Sarzi-Puttini et al., 2015). If left untreated, dysphagia can also have serious health-related consequences and a significant impact on quality of life. People with fibromyalgia who also have problems swallowing may be at even higher risk of psychosocial and overall health outcomes, yet little research has been carried out that explores the first-hand lived experience of people with fibromyalgia who have associated problems with eating, drinking and swallowing.

In order to go some way towards filling this gap in the existing literature, a study was carried out to explore the lived experience of people with fibromyalgia who are affected by oropharyngeal dysphagia and to identify any factors that may potentially influence the effect of their swallowing problems (Hussey & Gilheaney, 2022). The lived experience of the physical symptoms and the psychosocial impact of the symptoms were explored, as well as the strategies used by the participants to cope with the effects of having fibromyalgia and associated swallowing problems. Furthermore, the study also sought to identify the supporting strategies used by friends and family members to support their loved ones to live well.

Interviews were carried out with eight people who had fibromyalgia and related swallowing problems. Most of the participants were from the United Kingdom (n=7) and one participant was from the Republic of Ireland. The mean age of the participants was 55 with a range of 47–59. The recordings of the interviews were transcribed, and inductive thematic analysis was carried out on the narrative data to identify key themes (Braun & Clarke, 2021).

In relation to lived experience, two major themes were identified, focusing on social and emotional impact of fibromyalgia-associated dysphagia (Figure 3.1).

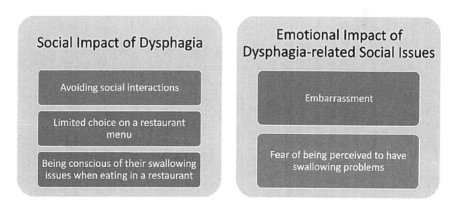

Figure 3.1 The social and emotional impact of fibromyalgia-associated dysphagia.

Major impacts of living with these swallowing problems included: avoiding social interactions, limited opportunities to dine out due to restricted diets, and being worried/conscious of swallowing issues when eating in company. Socialisation which involved eating and drinking (e.g., going out for a meal, meeting friends for drinks, etc.) was often avoided by participants, due either to suitable softer food choices not being on the menu, or to the worry that the person may have a frightening and embarrassing choking episode. The fear of choking has real life-limiting consequences that can take a social and emotional toll on people with fibromyalgia. This was illustrated by quotes such as:

> "I can't drink any alcohol. I can't enjoy life, particularly I can't go out for dinners."

and

> "When I go somewhere, I always explained to people look don't worry, I will cough and I might choke a bit, but it's part of my condition and I can't help it. I try not to, but you know, I'm sorry if I do and it upsets you or embarrasses you or whatever." (Hussey & Gilheaney, 2022).

Interestingly, these quotes from people with fibromyalgia from the UK and Ireland mirror comments by people living with fibromyalgia who contribute to global online support forums, suggesting a shared experience worldwide. For example, Gavigan and Gilheaney (2022) found that contributors to popular online support forums for fibromyalgia also experienced reduced choice when dining out, as a result of restrictive diets, e.g.,

> "Thank goodness for protein shakes. I have to order kids' meals everywhere I go or I will waste food."

In addition, anxiety related to choking has also been identified here as a major worry for people living with fibromyalgia-associated dysphagia:

> "I can have bits of food trapped in my esophagus for hours, unable to swallow or even drink water, and the only way to clear my throat is to induce vomiting repeatedly and cough it up bit by bit along with loads of mucus (sorry for the description). It's gotten bad enough to make me seriously afraid for my life."

These similar experiences suggest that these issues are common across countries and ethnicity of people living with fibromyalgia, highlighting the need for effective and empathetic support and management options.

As a result of reduced social opportunities, many people with fibromyalgia have also reported experiencing negative emotions associated with eating. The most common negative emotions reported in Hussey and Gilheaney (2022) were embarrassment and fear of social stigma associated with having swallowing problems, two concepts which are clearly interlinked. Embarrassment and shame regarding impaired swallowing was commonly reported, with participants becoming anxious that they may "cause a scene" in a restaurant if they had a choking episode. This led to them opting out of social situations where they may have had to eat in public, thereby leading them to avoid meeting with friends and family. This was demonstrated in quotes such as:

> "And I was so embarrassed because everybody was looking at me."

> "We went away a few weeks ago, and went to a fish restaurant. I ended up not finishing my meal, really because I was so scared of, you know, that I'm in a restaurant what if I end up choking."

> "I don't want to be causing a drama. I don't want, I would say I'm quite a I'm not a person that likes the spotlight. Like I'd rather just blend into the background."

> "I'm very conscious, because it's embarrassing, you know, I don't want to have a coughing fit, where I end up literally in tears from the choking, and you know, all your make-up washes down your face and you look like an imbecile, you know. So, it does it just limits life".

> "I'm always mortified if I have a choking fit."
> (Hussey & Gilheany, 2022).

On a more global scale, people living with fibromyalgia have also discussed their embarrassment about eating or drinking in public within online forums. These individuals have reported that they are embarrassed about the potential for overt symptoms of dysphagia occurring while they are eating or drinking in social settings (e.g., coughing, choking, regurgitation of food/fluid). For example:

> "Yeah, for me things always go down the wrong way making me have an almighty coughing fit! It's very embarrassing out in public as I also get bladder weakness and an asthma attack. It makes you feel so broken when things like that happen."

> "It drives me crazy and happens at pretty much every meal (like once or so a meal). It drives me batty."

> "Whenever I swallow food, I always feel it going down my esophagus the whole way because it gets stuck as it goes down and is very painful. I have to hit myself in the chest repeatedly to dislodge stuff and I don't even take large bites of food like it could literally be a single piece of shredded chicken or half a popcorn chicken nugget, etc."
> (Gavigan & Gilheaney, 2022).

Feeling anxious about choking when eating and drinking was the number one emotion reported by all participants of the study and the level of anxiety that they experienced ranged from a mild sense of worry to a severe fear of eating and drinking. The following quotations from participants of the study highlight the source and extent of anxiety and fear that is commonly felt by people with fibromyalgia and associated eating, drinking and swallowing problems:

> "And if I'm getting so anxious before I go out, I'm already not enjoying the experience because the anxiety is gone sky high cause I'm worrying about what I can order? What I can eat? Where the, the bathrooms are? Can I get there quick enough, you know, to finish coughing?"

> "It's quite frightening then because it feels like I can't breathe."

> "When I'm trying to eat something or when I'm thinking of going to eat something, I get really anxious, as to if I'm going to choke or not."

> "Sometimes even looking at an apple, I feel a bit anxious. Because I think last time I had that I choked."
> (Gavigan & Gilheaney, 2022.)

Self-doubt or self-blame was also a key theme identified in the narrative data from these studies. Participants questioned whether they themselves were at fault for their problems with swallowing. The following narrative extracts highlight the extent of self-doubt and self-blame that is commonly felt by people with fibromyalgia and associated swallowing problems:

> "So I don't know whether that's anything to do with that or if I'm drinking too fast or anything."

> "I was, blaming myself, I would be like, if I wasn't such a pig, now and ate a bit slower this mightn't happen."

> "It makes me feel like it makes me feel a bit useless to be honest. So then that kind of leads to a touch of, not depression, but it makes me feel it gets into my head that I'm not able to eat properly. I'm not able to do a lot of things with fibromyalgia. And it kind of makes me feel just a bit useless to be honest. If that makes sense."
> (Hussey & Gilheaney, 2022).

While some people may experience short-term or fluctuating swallowing problems in line with their overall fibromyalgia symptoms, others may experience more chronic and debilitating issues. Continual cancellation of social plans or avoidance of people with whom they were previously close, coupled with the general lack of awareness of invisible illnesses in the general public, may lead to narrowing of social circles over time. This narrowing of social circles can have a knock-on effect on a person's life, leading to feelings of isolation, and possibly depression (Pizzorni, 2017).

The fear of being perceived as having a swallowing problem often led participants to avoid situations where they would have to eat and drink in public. The following excerpts from participant interviews illustrate the nature and extent of the avoidance element of the social and emotional toll of having fibromyalgia and associated eating, drinking and swallowing problems:

> "...if I can, I would avoid going out to eat out. If I go shopping, I will just stop for a cup of tea. I won't normally have something with it. You know, like somebody'll have a nice little cake. It can be a tiny little crumb that sets it off."

> "So I have an avoidance personality."

> "It makes me feel like I don't want to go out for a meal. Going over to my son's house. I've got a grandson who lives

> with my son. And I'm not wanting to frighten them in case I start to choke." (Gavigan & Gilheaney, 2022).

Lack of enjoyment from food and feelings of self-doubt and self-blame when it comes to challenges with eating and drinking were also key themes identified in the analysis of data, as outlined below:

> "I can't drink any alcohol. I can't enjoy life, particularly I can't go out for dinners."

> "I'm eating to live I don't enjoy. I don't it's not an enjoyable experience to eat. I know I have to because I don't I won't survive without it."

> "There's been days when I haven't eaten anything."

> "It's horrible to think that I'm going to be like this forever. You know, it's because it's not very nice, and it's not very comfortable. And it there's no enjoyment out of food." (Gavigan & Gilheaney, 2022).

The key themes identified in the narrative data from these studies mirror the findings in the general dysphagia literature. The routine of daily living, for most people, is interspersed with social occasions that provide cognitive stimulation and meaningful interactions which enhance feelings of wellbeing; however, for people with dysphagia participation in these occasions is often curtailed as a result of their swallowing problem. Many of the occasions that give us pleasure and create memories centre around social eating. A qualitative systematic review of people with swallowing problems as a result of head and neck cancer was carried out by Dornan et al. (2021) and they identified the following two key social themes related to swallowing problems in the literature: "the loss of ability and confidence to eat and drink in a socially acceptable way" and "the experience of the loss of togetherness with family and friends" (p.4905). Meeting up with others to have a meal and share stories, tell a joke, have a laugh, and sometimes provide support when things aren't going as well as they could be, are important social facilitators of wellbeing. For people with swallowing problems, social occasions are greatly reduced as a result of the fear and anxiety they experience when they contemplate socialising with others at occasions where food and drink is part of the event (Farri, Accornero, & Burdese, 2007). Withdrawing from socialising can lead to an increase in social exclusion that negatively impacts on feelings of wellbeing and quality of life. Considering these findings, it is therefore not surprising that people with fibromyalgia-associated swallowing problems experience the same type of issues (Hussey & Gilheaney, 2022), yet the severity of these issues may be amplified secondary to their experience of the myriad of other primary symptoms (e.g., pain, fatigue, sleep, cognitive, and mood changes). Therefore, it is more important than ever that there is a growing awareness of these issues and their impact so that adequate supports and treatments can be put in place.

3.4 The complexity of fibromyalgia-associated dysphagia

Recent research suggests that the social and emotional consequences of dysphagia parallel, if not eclipse, the purely physical concerns. The different daily living challenges associated with the multiple symptoms of this disorder have a combined negative effect and create a large invisible obstacle that takes a toll on physical status, psychosocial health, and wellbeing.

4 Strategies for living well with fibromyalgia-associated dysphagia

Kathleen Mc Tiernan, Mathilde MacNamara
& Órla Gilheaney

4.1 The challenges of living with or caring for someone with a chronic illness

People living with chronic illness and their caregivers face similar challenges and can mutually benefit from learning about and using adaptive strategies to help them cope. These challenges and strategies are discussed in detail within this chapter, with a focus on developing and maintaining resilience and wellbeing.

4.2 Coping with swallowing problems

Participants in recent studies have reported using a range of independent and partner-assisted coping strategies in their attempt to live well with fibromyalgia-associated dysphagia. To begin, people with fibromyalgia have reported that they reduce the amount of food that they eat during the day and that they also restrict their diet by avoiding certain foods which are difficult to chew or swallow (e.g., apples, steak, baguettes, etc.) (Gavigan & Gilheaney, 2022; Hussey & Gilheaney, 2022). This coping strategy is reported to result in people often only eating a few select food items for all meals, despite potentially not being nutritionally optimal (e.g., dry crackers, yoghurts, ice cream) (Gavigan & Gilheaney, 2022). Despite these modifications, people with fibromyalgia have also discussed having to eat slowly, chew for a long time, and monitor their posture while eating so as to ensure swallow safety (Gavigan & Gilheaney, 2022). Participants in recent studies have also spoken about having to continuously drink while eating solids so as to "wash down" the food (Hussey & Gilheaney, 2022), with many participants depending on very hot or cold and carbonated/'fizzy' drinks to increase their sensory input (Gavigan & Gilheaney, 2022).

Notably, the majority of participants implemented various coping strategies, and with this independent self-management of symptoms came variable levels of success with participants reporting a significant amount of trial and error involved in their use. Researchers noted the potential dangers for people who self-modify or restrict their own diets without professional support, with the risk of malnutrition, unintentional weight changes, and dehydration, all of which would add to the baseline difficulties of living with fibromyalgia.

Participants in Gavigan and Gilheaney's study (2022) also reported that they often have to use self-soothing and calming techniques (e.g., deep breathing techniques) to maintain their composure and deal with unpleasant symptoms while eating and drinking. Participants often reported not eating when they were alone for fear of choking. In these cases, it was reported that friends and families of participants also promoted the use of such calming and relaxation strategies to help the person with fibromyalgia stay calm and continue their oral intake.

As outlined, much of the available research indicates that people with fibromyalgia typically manage their swallowing problems independently at home, relying on self-prescribed compensatory strategies, often with the help of friends or families who act as informal caregivers (MacNamara, 2022). This caregiving role has been described as primarily providing physical support (e.g., in the form of making specialised and modified meals or carrying out the Heimlich Manoeuvre when the person with fibromyalgia is choking on food) (Gavigan & Gilheaney, 2022; MacNamara, 2022) and emotional support (e.g., in promoting the use of relaxation strategies during meals:

Hussey & Gilheaney, 2022). These supports are often provided within the context of a friend or familial relationship, and individuals often report that they have accepted the role of caregiver and are happy to help their loved one (MacNamara, 2022).

However, the caring role is not without difficulties and caregivers have reported a range of negative emotions. Caregivers often report worry about their loved one choking and subsequently dying due to their swallowing issues. They also report that they often feel a sense of guilt if they cannot be present at all meals to ensure safe and supervised eating and drinking (MacNamara, 2022). This can lead to reduced participation in activities outside of the home and can further isolate both the person with fibromyalgia and their caregiver. In addition, frustration and anger with the fluctuation of dysphagia symptoms and the caregiver's own ability to improve the health of their loved one was common (MacNamara, 2022). Caregiver burden is evident, as social circles shrink and the person with fibromyalgia may often come to rely solely on their caregiver for all their needs without much outside support for themselves or, indeed, their caregiver (MacNamara, 2022).

4.3 General strategies for safe eating, drinking, and swallowing

Fibromyalgia-associated dysphagia has a broad range of possible symptoms and each person's illness profile is unique in presentation and impact. It can be challenging to provide specific guidance for a non-specific condition; however, despite this, there are a number of compensatory strategies which can improve the safety and effectiveness of eating, drinking, and swallowing, regardless of the underlying illness in question (Dorset HealthCare University NHS Foundation Trust, 2022; Nutricia, 2022; Reinstein, 2020). These tips do not replace the advice of a healthcare provider and the individual with dysphagia should always consult with their medical team before implementing new strategies. If there is an increase in swallowing problems, choking, coughing, a fever or breathing difficulties, the medical provider should be contacted immediately.

Figure 4.1 (overleaf) shows a number of tips and techniques. In addition to using these techniques, there are a number of healthcare professionals who, if consulted, can contribute to the multidisciplinary team (MDT) management of fibromyalgia-associated dysphagia (Logemann, 1994). These are itemised in Figures 4.2a and b (overleaf).

Posture and Behaviour

O Sit upright in a chair while you're eating and drinking - don't lie down if possible as this makes it difficult to swallow safely

O Stay upright for at least 30 minutes after every meal or drink to allow the materials to pass down into your stomach safely

O Don't talk while you are eating and drinking - you can breathe in food or drink and choke

O Eat in a comfortable and calm environment that makes you feel relaxed and doesn't have many distractions (e.g.: TV, radio)

O Maintain good oral hygiene by cleaning your mouth and teeth before and after each meal to avoid a build-up of residue.

Eating and Drinking Techniques

O Take small bites of food so that you have less to chew in each mouthful

O Take small sips of water instead of large gulps

O Sip water throughout a meal so as to wash down food

O Eat slowly and do not rush to swallow - this may make you chew the food less and put you at more risk of choking

O Make sure you have fully swallowed one mouthful before taking another

O Don't eat or drink while talking as you are more likely to breathe materials into your air pipe and have it "go the wrong way"

O Avoid using a straw if possible as these can send the drink back into your throat so quickly that you may not have time to control it safely

O Clear your mouth after eating to reduce your risk of coughing/choking on residue

Diet Modification

O Before you modify your food or drink, it is advisable to check in with a dietician and SLT to ensure that you can maintain optimal and safe nutrition and hydration

O Keep track of which foods and drinks are easy/hard to swallow and keep track of any trends or changes

O Be careful when eating mixed consistency foods (eg: stew that has soup and lumpy vegetables) as these can be difficult to swallow safely

O When eating really tough, crunchy, or stringy food, be sure to moisten it with sauce if appropriate, chew it for an extra-long time, and wash it down with a drink after you have swallowed it

Figure 4.1 General safe swallowing guidelines.

Health and Social Care Professionals
• **Speech and language therapist (SLT):** The SLT is a core member of the dysphagia multidisciplinary team. They contribute to management by identifying and assessing for signs and symptoms of dysphagia using a range of subjective assessments (e.g: bedside swallow exams) and objective tests (e.g: a videofluoroscopy or endoscopy), providing direct treatment for the issues underlying the dysphagia, advising on compensatory strategies to boost the safety of the swallow, measuring outcomes, and planning discharges. An important role of the SLT is educating and counselling people living with dysphagia and their caregivers about their dysphagia, the most appropriate food and fluid intake for swallow safety, and respecting decisions related to the patient's quality of life (The American Speech-Language-Hearing Association, 2022).
• **Dietician:** Dieticians can screen for dysphagia as part of a wider nutritional assessment. If you are taking a modified diet, the dietician can advise how to make it nutritionally optimal, including the use of nutritional supplements and/or alternative feeding methods if needed/appropriate (Macleod & O'Shea, 2019; Bordy et al., 2000).
• **Occupational therapist (OT):** OTs can assess and provide information on environmental and behavioural strategies to optimise swallow safety, while also advising on adapted mealtime set-up and appropriate equipment/cutlery and the best positioning for safe eating and drinking (The American Association of Occupational Therapists, 2011).
• **Physiotherapist (PT):** The PT can advise on optimal positioning and physical supports required to help the person with dysphagia to eat and drink safely. In addition, if the person with fibromyalgia-associated dysphagia develops a chest infection, the PT can provide chest physio (Godwin & Rogers, 2016).
• **Pharmacist:** Pharmacists are important team members as they can help to assess if medications that the person with fibromyalgia are taking are contributing to dysphagia (e.g: causing dry mouth). Additionally, the pharmacist can advise on if medications can be safely altered to make them easier to swallow (eg: by taking them in liquid versus solid form) (Stone, 2014; Wright, Begent & Crawford, 2017).

Figure 4.2a Multidisciplinary healthcare professionals who can contribute to the management of fibromyalgia-associated dysphagia.

Medical, Surgical and Nursing Professionals

●**General practitioner (GP):** The GP can help with initial detection and management of dysphagia, while also ensuring that you are referred onto the other relevant team members for further investigation (NHS, 2022).

●**Gastroenterologist:** The gastroenterologist can contribute to diagnosis by determining if a swallowing problem is caused by the oropharyngeal or oesophageal muscles. They can do so using tests like a barium swallow, high-resolution manometry or endoscopy and can contribute to the medical management of oesophageal dysphagia (Hollenbach et al., 2018).

●**Otolaryngologist:** If the dysphagia is caused by a problem at the oropharngeal stage, the otolaryngologist can contribute to diagnosis by conducting a laryngoscope or endoscope. They can also contribute to both the medical and surgical management of dysphagia, if apporpriate (Duval et al., 2009).

●**Neurologist:** Dysphagia can result from problems with your nerves, the brain itself, or the spinal cord. In this case, the neurologist can aid with diagnosis through clinical and objective assessments and help to plan the most effective management in the overall context of the patient's presenting condition, prognosis, and level of disability (Hughes & Wiles, 1998).

●**Pulmonologist:** Dysphagia can result due to incoordination between the swallowing and breathing mechanisms caused by common respiratory conditions (e.g: chronic obstructive pulmonary disorder). Also, if you breathe in bits of food and drink (aspiration), you can develop a chest infection. The pulmonologist can help to diagnose and treat these respiratory conditions and can work together with other team members to maximise respiratory health (McKinstry, Tranter & Sweeney, 2010; Ghannouchi et al., 2016; Lillie et al., 2014).

●**Radiologist:** Radiologists have a role in imaging the head and neck anatomy and swallow mechanism through scans such as the videofluoroscopy or barium swallow. This can help contribute to diagnosis and help judge how effective management strategies have been (Grant et al., 2009; Ghazanfar et al., 2021).

●**Registered Nurse:** Nurses have an important role in screening for swallowing problems to contribute to early detection, in addition to supporting the overall management of dysphagia (Abu-Snieneh & Saleh, 2018).

Figure 4.2b Multidisciplinary healthcare professionals who can contribute to the management of fibromyalgia-associated dysphagia.

It is important to remember that, regardless of the number of clinicians listed, the most important members of the clinical team are always the person living with fibromyalgia-associated dysphagia and their loved ones/caregivers as they are the true experts in these issues (Farneti & Consolmagno, 2007).

4.4 Living with chronic illness

The difficulties associated with living with dysphagia are not confined to simply the mechanics of swallowing. There are also challenges to the psychosocial wellbeing of people living with swallowing difficulties and their caregivers. The research on wellbeing and resilience (Kim, Lim, Kim, & Park, 2019) for those living with chronic illness is applicable here as these strategies may facilitate people with fibromyalgia-associated dysphagia and their caregivers to maintain positive social, emotional, and functional well-being, despite the daily challenges that they face.

Enduring a prolonged episode of pain or going through a particularly difficult time for any reason can lead to feelings of being overwhelmed and exhausted and these can lead to a reduction in attention to basic daily living needs (Figure 4.3). Neglecting basic daily living needs can have a negative emotional effect on one's overall sense of wellbeing (Stoewen, 2017; White, Issac, Kamoun, Leygues, & Cohn, 2018).

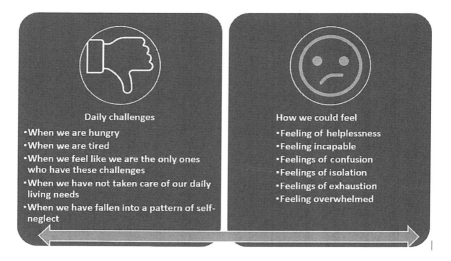

Figure 4.3 Emotional consequences of common daily challenges.

Long-term experience of physically and/or emotionally demanding situations can lead to feelings of physical and mental exhaustion or 'burnout'. There are a number of practical adaptive behaviours that have been proven to help us feel physically and emotionally better, even when going through a particularly challenging set of circumstances (Figure 4.4).

Creating adaptive habits can have a significant positive impact on the overall sense of wellbeing. By attending to daily living needs, even by changing one or two small daily living practices, we can greatly influence our quality of life and wellbeing (Gardner, Lally, & Wardle, 2012; Stojanovic, Fries, & Grund, 2021).

So far in this chapter we have discussed the many ways that people with fibromyalgia and associated swallowing problems can bolster their physical and psychosocial wellbeing. It is important to remember that caregivers and family members who are in caring roles can also be affected by the physical and psychosocial challenges associated with caring for someone with a chronic condition (Sullivan & Miller, 2015). Many of the methods for enhancement

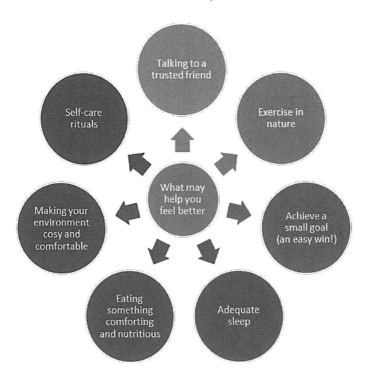

Figure 4.4 Small actions which may help those living with chronic illness to feel better.

of physical and emotional wellbeing mentioned here are directly applicable to family and caregivers of people with chronic illnesses.

Some of the challenges that caregivers face may include feelings of isolation, the changing relationship with a loved one, and neglecting their own physical, social and emotional needs (Irfan, Irfan, Ansari, Qidwai, & Nanji, 2017). Furthermore, caregivers often report that they do not have enough time for self-care and this can lead to a habitual pattern of self neglect as they repeatedly put the needs of the person that they are caring for ahead of their own needs (Irfan et al., 2017). Often many of the same needs that caregivers meet for the people that they care for can be the same self-care needs that they are neglecting for themselves. Time management is often difficult for caregivers and finding a balance between the demands of a caregiving role and their own self-care needs is challenging. Caregivers may benefit from a referral to mental health or medical services in order to address some of the strain on their own mental and physical health that often goes along with a caregiving role (Sullivan & Miller, 2015).

4.5 Health beliefs, self-care, and collaborative care

Self-care and having a coping perspective are important elements that help people with chronic conditions and their caregivers thrive over time (Hawken, Turner-Cobb, & Barnett, 2018). We all have health beliefs, or ways of thinking about our own health, and caregivers and family members also have their own health beliefs that may be different from ours. Individual health beliefs are related to several factors including: demographics (age, gender, race, socioeconomics, etc.), perceived threat of health condition, perceived benefit of treatment or action and perceived self-efficacy or control (Ogden, 2019). Understanding that individual health beliefs shape how we cope and self-manage fibromyalgia-related dysphagia can be an important step in adapting our lifestyles so that we prioritise self-care.

It is important to be aware that approaches to chronic health conditions often differ and that conflicting health beliefs can have a negative impact on both self and collaborative management of chronic illnesses. Understanding that people have different health beliefs is an important factor in conflict management within a caregiving dynamic (Marín-Maicas et al., 2021). Knowing that we may have fundamentally different health beliefs is the key to understanding why approaches to management and care differ. The knowledge that we all have individual health beliefs can empower us to learn from each other and communicate our needs and goals more effectively (Rowe et al., 2019). Accepting that people often view chronic illness from different underlying health belief perspectives is the first step in developing collaborative care plans with caregivers and/or family members (Martire & Helgeson, 2017). Preserving respectful relationships that value individual differences and working together to meet healthcare and lifestyle goals is ultimately what people with chronic conditions and their caregivers and/or family strive to achieve.

4.6 Links between thoughts, feelings and behaviours

In the same way that changing one or two practical daily living practices can have the knock-on effect of interrupting negative emotions, changing a minor aspect of our patterns of thinking can also have a significant impact on how we feel about and react to life's challenges (Fenn & Byrne, 2013). Thoughts frame our behaviours and our behaviours frame our thoughts, and by changing either one of these the other changes too.

This is not to say that we can change how we think and as a result all our challenges will go away, however, there is no doubt that practising adaptive thinking can help us cope with life's challenges (Büssing et al., 2010). Creating a routine of thinking, that allows for the mental space to take a moment of pause between stimulus and response, can create a greater sense of control, can put us back in the driver's seat and can enable us to make choices and decisions that perhaps we would not have considered in the absence of taking the time to collect our thoughts and consider our options. In order to explore how to implement some of the techniques mentioned here, seeking a referral to a registered mental health professional may be a useful first step to take on the journey to increasing physical and psychosocial wellbeing while living with a chronic illness.

4.7 The importance of supporting both the person living with fibromyalgia-associated dysphagia and their caregivers

The challenges for people with chronic illness and the associated challenges for their loved ones who are providing care are numerous. Adaptive strategies and suggested coping mechanisms to alleviate some of the physical and psychosocial impact of having fibromyalgia-associated dysphagia that are provided here are equally applicable for both the person with the dysphagia and those providing them with support. Implementing even one or two of the strategies suggested here can improve wellbeing and health outcomes. The next chapter outlines enablers and barriers to the provision of professional healthcare to this group of people, incorporating research, clinician views, and patient accounts.

5 How can healthcare professionals support people with fibromyalgia-associated dysphagia?

Órla Gilheaney, Ellen Carroll & Kathleen Mc Tiernan

5.1 The provision of healthcare for people with fibromyalgia-associated dysphagia

This chapter presents a thorough account of the research regarding the provision of healthcare for people with fibromyalgia-associated dysphagia. Information has been collated from the existing research in this field, practising clinicians, and firsthand patient experiences to describe the enablers and barriers to the provision of best practice healthcare for people with fibromyalgia-associated dysphagia.

5.2. Current healthcare provision: The practice and perspectives of clinicians

Despite many people with fibromyalgia-associated swallowing difficulties living well, independently and with the support provided by their caregivers, some patients have to look beyond this support and seek out professional healthcare support to address their severe eating, drinking, and swallowing problems. To date, research has documented the difficulties that patients have faced when seeking professional care for fibromyalgia-associated dysphagia (Hussey & Gilheaney, 2022). For example: due to their already long and varied list of primary symptoms, patients have reported being reluctant to report additional swallowing issues to healthcare providers because clinicians are already busy focusing on managing their existing challenges (Gavigan & Gilheaney, 2022). Unfortunately, some people with fibromyalgia have reported feeling unheard when they do report their dysphagia. While this is certainly not always the case, as there are accounts of supportive therapeutic relationships in the literature, some patients report feeling dismissed after telling clinicians about their swallowing difficulties (e.g., "all in your head") (Gavigan & Gilheaney, 2022; Hussey & Gilheaney, 2022). It may well be the case that some clinicians do not recognise that fibromyalgia can be associated with dysphagia. However, a mismatch in patient-clinician priorities can impact negatively on satisfaction with care, leading to avoidance of future care-seeking opportunities which may pose a risk to patient wellbeing (Gavigan & Gilheaney, 2022; Hussey & Gilheaney, 2022).

The impact of this is not only felt by patients but also by their loved ones and caregivers (MacNamara, 2022). Caregivers have reported that they feel a lack of support and understanding from some clinicians regarding the swallowing issues that their loved ones are living with. In addition, research shows that when caregivers seek education or training on how best to support their loved one, adequate resources are often not available to provide guidance (MacNamara, 2022).

Research suggests that many healthcare professionals also feel similarly uncertain and unsupported when working with people with fibromyalgia-associated dysphagia (Carroll, Mc Tiernan, & Gilheaney, 2022). A recent scoping review has shown that clinicians face many barriers when providing care to people living with dysphagia and chronic pain conditions (e.g., fibromyalgia) due to the lack of clinical guidelines and treatment options, leading to unmet medical needs within this group (Flanagan & Gilheaney, 2022). Carroll et al. (2022) recently surveyed international healthcare practitioners about their current practice patterns, attitudes, and beliefs about the assessment and management of eating and drinking problems in people living with fibromyalgia. A range of professionals participated in the survey, including SLTs, neurologists, physiotherapists, occupational therapists, and dieticians. Participants reported limited experience with people with fibromyalgia-related swallowing issues, with a third of participants reporting that they never enquire about or assess for these problems, and two-thirds reporting that they never provide treatment for these concerns. Clinicians who do assess patients for these challenges typically rely on the following methods of evaluation: case history, orofacial exams, swallow screening tools, clinical swallow exams, or objective assessments. More than a quarter of participants reported referring patients onwards to other clinicians for assessment purposes. When treatment was provided, it most often took the form of patient education, compensatory strategies, diet modifications, liaison with multidisciplinary colleagues, onward referral, and medication adjustment (Carroll et al., 2022).

Notably, although most clinicians in this study reported feeling a lack of confidence about working with people living with fibromyalgia and swallowing problems, qualitative data suggested that the clinicians surveyed were aware of patient concerns regarding stigma and were therefore cautious not to dismiss their symptoms and to acknowledge and honour their illness experience, e.g.:

> "I have witnessed fibromyalgia patients being brushed aside as hypochondriacs and getting minimal interests from care providers." (Carroll et al., 2022).

Clinicians often attributed their uncertainty and lack of confidence to the lack of awareness, resources, research, and practical guidance for clinicians working in this field to provide the best practice care and support to their patients (Carroll et al., 2022).

Furthermore, this study also found that clinicians wished to learn more about their professional role and responsibility with this group so that they could optimise their care delivery to this group. Therefore, despite the uncertainty of both patients and clinicians regarding optimal service provision, both parties want to improve their knowledge of the condition and its management, with the ultimate goal of improving patient outcomes and wellbeing.

5.3 Future directions for optimal provision of care

Discussions at the public FibroForum conference in Trinity College Dublin (https://fibroforumtcd.online/) suggested that the needs of both patients and clinicians are very similar with regards to care provision for fibromyalgia-associated dysphagia (Gilheaney & McTiernan, 2022). Participants at the FibroForum reported that they all saw the need to strengthen the therapeutic alliance between clinicians and patients (Gilheaney & McTiernan, 2022) which resembles what clinicians reported in the study by Carroll and colleagues (2022). However, while clinicians in this study were often unsure of how to achieve this goal, contributors to the Fibroforum who live with fibromyalgia-associated dysphagia offered a range of suggestions

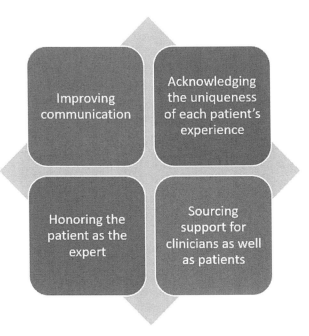

Figure 5.1 Possible future developments in health provision.

for future developments in care provision. Themes which were identified from analysis of contributor comments are outlined in Figure 5.1.

5.3.1 Improving patient-clinician communication

Improving communication between professionals and patients was flagged as an area for future development in care provision to people living with fibromyalgia-associated dysphagia. This is notable as improved communication between clinicians and patients has been previously identified as essential to the provision of high-quality medical care, regardless of the patient cohort (Davis, 2010). People living with fibromyalgia-associated dysphagia acknowledged that, while *"fibro is hard to explain"*, clinicians should strive to use accessible, 'patient friendly' language and actively listen to their experiences in an effort to understand their perspectives. Several contributors reported appreciating when clinicians communicate in a straightforward and transparent way, talking *"to people as people"* and *"speaking to the human being"* as opposed to using overly formal medical jargon. Finally, attendees at the FibroForum reported that they also value clinicians who were more *"collaborative with patients"* in care planning and decision making (Gilheaney & McTiernan, 2022).

These patient perspectives mirror findings from literature where, historically, the majority of medical complaints relate to breakdowns in communication as opposed to a lack of clinical competency (Richards, 1990). Communication issues usually relate to use of medical jargon, a lack of listening to patients and hearing their needs, and minimal transparency and shared ownership in decision making. All of these factors can negatively affect interactions, commitment to and perceptions of treatments, and health outcomes (Meryn, 1998; Neeman et al., 2012).

Research has shown that there are correlations between effective clinician communication and improved patient outcomes (Stewart, 1995). Communication is especially challenging when an illness is invisible and has a myriad of associated concerns, like in the case of fibromyalgia (Fong & Longnecker, 2010). Communication mismatches can lead to a difference in clinician and patient perceptions and expressed views about the nature of the problem, the goals of treatment, and prognosis. This can result in a breakdown in communication and trust (Fong & Longnecker, 2010). It is essential that communication between clinicians and patients is empathetic in order to facilitate transparent sharing of information, accurate identification of patient needs, expectations, and priorities, and to ensure satisfaction with care provided.

To improve communication, clinicians and patients can focus on relationship-building from the very first meeting, by using active listening skills, displaying empathy, and involving each other in the co-construction of a shared narrative. This can be achieved by providing written and verbal information, by using open-ended questioning, by checking in regularly regarding each other's understanding of the key issues and information, and by involvement of patients and significant others in decision making (Brédart, Bouleuc, & Dolbeault, 2005; Fong & Longnecker, 2010; Gulbrandsen, 2020). By using accessible language and actively working to seek to understand perspectives and unique health beliefs, potential conflicts can be minimised and managed effectively (Neeman et al., 2012; Tongue, Epps, & Forese, 2005).

Research has indicated that, over time, some clinicians can become burned out, further impacting their communication skills (Fong & Longnecker, 2010). It has been suggested that in cases such as this, active continuing professional development and skill-based peer-group improvement activities can be beneficial to improving baseline communication skills in order to augment patient satisfaction and outcomes into the future (Belasen & Belasen, 2018a; Belasen & Belasen, 2018b; Hobma et al., 2006; Korzh & Tsodikova, 2019; Kurtz, 2002; McCabe & Healey, 2018).

5.3.2 Honouring the unique patient journey and their lived experience and expertise

Comments from attendees at the FibroForum (Gilheaney & McTiernan, 2022) about their priorities for optimal healthcare centred on two similar themes: the importance of acknowledging patients as experts in living with fibromyalgia-associated dysphagia and understanding that their unique lived experiences and journeys can enrich our understanding of the illness. Historically, the value of patient lived experience has sometimes been overlooked, with narrative accounts not being valued as core components of understanding the nature, prognosis, and reality of living with a chronic illness (Donaldson, 2003). However, the recent move away from a medical model of healthcare towards a more consumer-led model of shared decision making and collaborative communication has highlighted the need to seek and emphasise patients' unique wisdom and expertise (Arora, 2003; Fong & Longnecker, 2010; Herndon & Pollick, 2002; Kindler et al., 2005). Attendees at the FibroForum (Gilheaney & McTiernan, 2022) reported that they believe that it is essential for clinicians to

> "hear from patients as we are experts",

reporting that clinicians should also

> "understand the [patients] value [as] the patient is [their] best evidence".

Actively listening to, and truly hearing, the stories of people living with chronic illness can give clinicians new insights into what living with a chronic condition is really like. As such, there are obvious benefits of truly validating and collaborating with patients for the clinician-patient relationship, patient wellbeing, and satisfaction with care. However, beyond these factors, person-centred care can also help identify previously unknown needs and priorities, thus positively shaping future research and treatment options (Cordier, 2014). This can then lead to improved engagement with and use of healthcare services, in addition to enhancing patient outcomes.

5.3.3 Support for clinicians to deal with isolation and uncertainty

Following on from the discussion above, it is also important to address the clinical isolation and uncertainty that many healthcare professionals report when working with patients living with chronic illnesses (Kim & Lee, 2018), especially among those experiencing under-researched and invisible illnesses. As participants in the FibroForum (Gilheaney & McTiernan, 2022) reported *"Although clinicians have a lack of knowledge, maybe there is none to be found"* and that this uncertainty can *"put a strain on a professional relationship"*. Acknowledging and addressing this isolation and uncertainty can be the first step in improving trust and balance in patient-clinician relationships. This could ultimately improve patient outcomes, and in addition it can enhance the professional job satisfaction of those working with people experiencing fibromyalgia-associated dysphagia (Kim & Lee, 2018).

Research suggests that technical uncertainty in medicine arises when there is limited evidence about a condition or its treatment (Beresford, 1991), such as in fibromyalgia-associated dysphagia. However, this lack of clarity can then be worsened by personal uncertainty whereby there is a breakdown in communication between a patient and clinician, leading to mutual isolation. Often this breakdown happens because clinicians struggle to apply the limited data about a certain illness to the complex realities of patients' struggles (Kim & Lee, 2018). Interestingly, research has shown that clinicians who have higher levels of stress due to clinical uncertainty experience poorer mental health, greater levels of work-related burnout and stress, and poorer work-related satisfaction (Bachman & Freeborn, 1999; Bovier & Perneger, 2007; Iannello et al., 2017). It has been suggested that clinicians may perceive uncertainty as a threat. Therefore, 'complex' patients who bring that uncertainty into the clinic may also be inadvertently viewed as a threat, leading to clinician uncertainty and a lack of confidence in interacting with the patient (Hillen et al., 2017). This can be damaging to the healthcare relationship which is central to all successful treatments.

There have been positive strategies reported for dealing with medical uncertainty which can improve clinicians' interactions with patients with complex needs, and therefore improve the overall clinical experience and outcomes. For example, Hillen and colleagues (2017) suggested approaching the uncertainty directly, seeking more information through a range of channels, with subsequent action and decision making as strategies for confronting and reducing uncertainty. Farnan et al. (2008) also suggested the need for a supervisory structure which was open, curious, and did not punish knowledge gaps when clinicians sought information or help from their colleagues or superiors. It is also suggested that supervision or support can be sought from clinical networks, special interest groups, or research institutions who are investigating these topics. In line with the discussion above, Ghosh (2004) emphasised the need to involve the patient themselves in acknowledging uncertainty and decision making, so as to strengthen trust as the basis of relationship building. Cristancho et al. (2013) reported that, when positive actions such as those listed above became staples of clinical practice, professionals became more tolerant of uncertainty over time and felt less isolated. Patients are unique and complex individuals, living varied and rich lives, which naturally differ from one another and will not fit the 'one size fits all' template (Helou et al., 2020). As such, it is essential that clinicians become more aware and tolerant of uncertainty and ensure that it does not damage their own effectiveness in their post, or the experience of their patients.

5.4 Embracing facilitators of optimal care provision

Although there are currently a number of obstacles to the optimal provision of care to this group, it is clear that by embracing the facilitators outlined by the practising clinicians and patient accounts discussed here, healthcare providers can begin to take the necessary steps towards the provision of effective and compassionate care. The next chapter summarises our exploration of fibromyalgia-associated dysphagia and provides final guidance on living with this condition and healthcare provision and research conducted within this field of study.

6 The future of collaborative care provision and research into fibromyalgia-associated dysphagia

Órla Gilheaney & Kathleen Mc Tiernan

6.1 The next steps in service delivery, clinical research, and policy development

Over the course of this book, we have presented a holistic account of the physical and psychosocial impact of fibromyalgia-associated dysphagia, drawing on recent research and firsthand accounts of patient experiences. In addition, we have highlighted the importance of caring for oneself and others in an empathetic, compassionate, and evidence-based way. In this chapter we summarise the key findings and messages from the previous chapters, re-emphasise links to the seminal literature in the area, and provide information regarding the recommended next steps in service delivery, clinical research, and policy development to advance understanding and care provision in this area. These recommendations will be consistently presented through the lens of promoting collaboration and co-construction of research priorities, plans, and findings between patients, their loved ones, clinicians, academics, and other relevant stakeholders. This process is commonly known as 'patient and public involvement' in research (PPI). This approach evidences the need to prioritise patients' lived experience, in addition to honouring patients' and their loved ones' concerns and priorities within research plans. PPI is becoming more common in research that creates and maintains active and mutually enriching relationships among researchers, clinicians, and academics to ensure that research and development reflects the true needs of those living with the health condition (Rouleau et al., 2018; Smith, Bélise-Pipon & Resnik, 2019). This chapter highlights the key role that PPI plays in optimal patient empowerment, excellent care provision, and meaningful positive outcomes.

6.2 Redefining fibromyalgia-associated dysphagia

Swallowing difficulties are rarely mentioned in relation to fibromyalgia in published academic literature. However, we still believe it is vital to investigate this topic further due to the myriad of anecdotal patient reports about the eating and swallowing difficulties that they often experience while living with fibromyalgia (Gavigan & Gilheaney, 2022). These issues include: trouble chewing solids, coughing while drinking fluids, pain on eating and swallowing, and dry mouth, among other concerns. Furthermore, Hussey & Gilheaney (2022) and Gavigan and Gilheaney (2022) emphasised the significant social and emotional impact of these eating and drinking problems, with reduced levels of socialisation, swallowing- and choking-related fear and shame, and self-doubt and blame.

Although research has not yet established a definitive cause for fibromyalgia-associated dysphagia, there have been tentative suggestions regarding the role of central sensitisation, polypharmacy, co-occurring structural, neurological and immunological issues, and fatigue-related concerns. Patient accounts regarding these experiences are readily accessible online (Gavigan & Gilheaney, 2022) and are also echoed in a small number of patient-focused studies (Hussey & Gilheaney, 2022). As the recognition of fibromyalgia-associated dysphagia gains recognition with the publication of research in this field, patients and clinicians both still report being unsure regarding the best methods of managing these concerns (Carroll et al., 2022; Gavigan & Gilheaney, 2022; Hussey & Gilheaney, 2022). Therefore, the exploration of this topic highlighting expert patient voices with firsthand experience of their symptoms is both timely and essential.

As this is an emerging research area, it is important to restate that we are still learning about the prevalence, nature, and impact of fibromyalgia-associated dysphagia. However, this book synthesises the current published work in the area and provides a solid foundation for subsequent explorations of eating and swallowing problems for people with fibromyalgia. There is clearly a lot more work to be done in this area and the inclusion of those living with and caring for those with fibromyalgia-associated dysphagia is vital in ensuring that patient voices and priorities are honoured and service delivery is optimised in the future.

6.3 Caring for yourself and others living with fibromyalgia-associated dysphagia

As our understanding of fibromyalgia-associated dysphagia increases, the ethical impetus to provide guidance for those living with or caring for those who experience these issues is also raised. As outlined in Chapter 4, there is currently a lack of knowledge regarding management strategies specifically designed for this cohort. This is due to the lack of clarity regarding the true underlying cause of fibromyalgia-associated dysphagia. We can, however, draw on common principles of general management for those living with other swallowing and chronic health difficulties, and advise on broad compensatory, supportive, and protective strategies as an interim measure.

6.3.1 Patient-directed eating and drinking strategies

People living with fibromyalgia-associated swallowing problems often report using compensatory strategies to deal with specific dysphagia symptoms. Due to the lack of clinical or research guidance in this area, these strategies are often used on a trial-and-error basis, with individuals developing unique coping habits (of varying effectiveness) by necessity, and often turning to online communities for inspiration and support. These strategies often centre on changes in eating habits and oral intake (e.g., eating less food or eating only softer and more processed food) and changes in swallowing techniques (e.g., excessive chewing or slower eating). While these strategies may immediately ease eating and drinking problems in the moment, they can lead to more long-term issues when used without clinical guidance. These issues can include increased pain and fatigue while chewing and swallowing, resulting in meal abandonment and adverse nutritional effects (e.g., unintentional weight loss, or malnutrition). Although investigators are currently exploring condition-specific solutions, there is a need for immediate support for those living with these issues.

A range of compensatory strategies were suggested earlier to alleviate moment-by-moment symptoms of swallowing difficulties among this group. These include generalised postural and behavioural strategies, a range of potentially helpful eating and drinking techniques, and cautious diet modification guidelines. As mentioned, these techniques should be used in conjunction with professional guidance, and the breadth of potential cross-disciplinary involvement in an ideal MDT was discussed. In Chapter 4, we outlined the need for medical, dental, allied health, and nursing involvement in order to fully support patients and their loved ones to live well despite fibromyalgia-associated dysphagia. It is essential to reiterate that all patient care must be guided by patient priorities and lived experiences in order to ensure that research findings are impactful in a real-life context.

6.3.2 Patient-directed strategies for living well with chronic health concerns

Going beyond specific eating and drinking strategies, people with chronic illnesses, including those living with fibromyalgia-associated swallowing problems, often have additional daily living stressors that they have to manage. Therefore nurturing and self-care activities are often pushed down the agenda as more pressing daily living needs take priority. Highlighting the need and providing support for self-care is an important element of patient-centred management of chronic illness (Kennedy et al., 2007). Table 6.1 displays a short list of some of the resources about self-care for people with a range of chronic illnesses that are freely available online at the time of publication.

6.3.3 Caregiver-directed strategies for living well when caring for others with chronic health concerns

When discussing chronic illness care, the focus is more often than not on the patient care and not much thought is given to the need for caregivers to care for themselves. A shift in healthcare providers' focus from the patient with the chronic illness to the caregiver is sometimes an important step in the provision of holistic care (Sherman et al., 2016). A number of negative health consequences can be associated with caring for a family member with a chronic illness and it is important for healthcare professionals to highlight to caregivers the importance of practising self-care and seeking support for themselves. Caregivers are often so focused on the needs of the recipients of

Table 6.1 Examples of informal self-care resources for people with chronic illnesses.

Resource example	Website link
Tips for self-care for people with fibromyalgia	**Fibromyalgia Self-Care Tips. (2019). Ruben Castaneda.** Access at: https://health.usnews.com/conditions/fibromyalgia/fibromyalgia-tips
Living well with fibromyalgia	**Living Well With Fibromyalgia. (2021). Julie Canter.** Access at: https://www.webmd.com/fibromyalgia/guide/living-with-fibromyalgia-tips
Self-love and self-care	**Self-Love and Self-Care: What Chronic Illness Taught Me About Both. (2021). Eileen Davidson.** Access at: https://creakyjoints.org/about-arthritis/rheumatoid-arthritis/ra-patient-perspectives/self-care-self-love-chronic-illness/
Learning to pace yourself	**Learning to Pace Myself. (2022). Eileen Davidson.** Access at: https://creakyjoints.org/about-arthritis/rheumatoid-arthritis/ra-patient-perspectives/learning-to-pace-myself/
The Spoon Theory and self-care	**I'm a "Spoonie." Here's What I Wish More People Knew About Chronic Illness. (2019). Kirsten Schultz.** Access at: https://www.healthline.com/health/spoon-theory-chronic-illness-explained-like-never-before#1
Tips to save energy and stress for parents with chronic illnesses	**Have You Been Budgeting Your Spoons This School Year? (2022). Stefanie Remson.** Access at: https://creakyjoints.org/about-arthritis/rheumatoid-arthritis/ra-patient-perspectives/budgeting-spoons-this-school-year/ Have You Been Budgeting Your Spoons This School Year?

their care that they neglect their own health and self-care needs (Sullivan & Miller, 2015). There are many useful websites, like the ones listed below, that provide an overview of simple ways in which carers can practice self-care in their daily lives. Table 6.2 displays a short list of some online resources about self-care for caregivers of people with chronic illnesses.

When caregivers are so focused on ensuring that care recipients' daily living needs are met they often neglect themselves in the process. Prioritising self-care is paramount for caregivers as they cannot provide care for another person if they are not attending to their own daily living needs.

Table 6.2 Examples of informal self-care resources for caregivers of people with chronic illnesses.

Resource Examples	Website link
Self-care for the caregiver	**Self-care for the Caregiver. (2018). Marlynn Wei.** Access at: https://www.health.harvard.edu/blog/self-care-for-the-caregiver-2018101715003
Caregiver stress: Tips for taking care of yourself	**Caregiver Stress: Tips for Taking Care of Yourself. (2022). Mayo Clinic Staff.** Access at: https://www.mayoclinic.org/healthy-lifestyle/stress-management/in-depth/caregiver-stress/art-20044784
Self-care for caregivers	**Self-Care for Caregivers. (2022). The Regents of The University of California.** Access at: https://www.ucsfhealth.org/education/self-care-for-caregivers
Taking care of yourself: Self-care for family caregivers	**Taking Care of YOU: Self-Care for Family Caregivers. (2022). The Family Caregiver Alliance.** Access at: https://www.caregiver.org/resource/taking-care-you-self-care-family-caregivers/
Caregiver self-care booklet: A guide to caregiver self-care	**A Guide To Caregiver Self-Care. (2019). Mary Catherine Lundquist et al.** Access at: https://www.care2caregivers.com/wp-content/uploads/2019/12/Caregiver-Self-Care-Booklet-English.pdf

6.4 The future of healthcare provision for people living with fibromyalgia-associated dysphagia

There is a range of care and research priorities which must be addressed to improve service delivery and optimal outcomes of people living with fibromyalgia-associated dysphagia. While we have reviewed the experiences and priorities of patients and their loved ones above, it is also essential that clinicians are part of the PPI process in the future. Professionals have reported feeling under-prepared to effectively support this group, leading to frustration and unmanaged uncertainty (Carroll et al., 2022; Flanagan & Gilheaney, 2022). Similar difficulties have been outlined in previous research which show that clinicians face a number of challenges in providing care to patients with chronic illnesses. These challenges include: (1) organisational barriers (e.g., time constraints or staff shortages); (2) interpersonal barriers (e.g., lack of knowledge regarding the importance of relationship building); and (3) individual barriers (e.g., lack of belief in the patient's lived experience) (Grilo et al., 2017). These factors can make it difficult for clinicians to implement effective patient-centred care.

Patients and clinicians have shared priorities, including relationship building and strengthening, improvement of patient-professional communication, and collaborative decision-making. These core priorities mirror the fundamental principles of patient-centred care, such as: understanding, acknowledging and legitimising the patient experience; developing and iteratively strengthening collaborative relationships; offering realistic hope; and advocating for increased awareness of and services for patients living with chronic health concerns (Grilo et al., 2017). Research has suggested that when the lived experience of the patient is central to the patient-clinician relationship, clinical outcomes are optimised. Some specific strategies to achieve these goals are discussed below.

6.4.1 Improved communication

The key to leveraging a shared vision of patient-centred care, that leads to improved quality of life and increased participation in all life domains, is establishing clear lines of communication between patients, caregivers and healthcare professionals. Articulating a shared vision with open, honest, respectful communication is transformative. It can be challenging, however, to establish these clear lines of communication. People with fibromyalgia-related swallowing problems may feel that, although they are the ones actually living with the problem, they are not always heard by those who are caring for them. Accepting help can be challenging for people with chronic illnesses like fibromyalgia and there may be an inclination to try to 'go it alone' as it can be difficult to admit the need for support. Healthcare professionals can sometimes feel that they know what is best for patients and they may proceed with plans of action without sufficient consultation with patients and caregivers. Caregivers can often feel out of the loop and overwhelmed and their views may not be given due consideration by those receiving their care or by healthcare professionals. All of the stakeholders, because of the pressures that are unique to their roles, may take communication shortcuts which can lead to patterns of negative interaction lacking the necessary collaborative features of patient-centred care. Although patients, healthcare professionals and caregivers may feel that the communication difficulties that they experience are unique to their particular situation, they are not uncommon and there are a number of resources available that acknowledge the issues related to communication within the patient centred care framework. Table 6.3 displays a short list of some of the useful communication resources which are available online.

6.4.2 Shared decision making and problem solving

Having a chronic illness, or being a healthcare provider/caregiver of a person with a chronic illness can be stressful. Developing a problem-solving mindset is an essential ingredient when establishing positive stakeholder relationships that can reduce stress levels for all involved. The key ingredients of collaborative problem solving is recognising that the patient is the expert in their own illness experience and utilising patient expertise in the treatment and management of chronic pain and illness will lead to optimal treatment outcomes. Patient participation in the decision-making process leads to improved health outcomes and an increase in patient empowerment (Birkeland et al., 2022). Helping patients take charge of their own chronic illnesses and leveraging patient expertise in the lived experience of chronic conditions informs collaborative healthcare decisions, and it should be the lens through which all health and care decisions are made. Historically, healthcare has been physician-directed and patients were passive recipients of care. More and more, however, healthcare professionals and people with chronic health conditions are moving toward a healthcare model that places the patient at the centre of the decision-making process. This shared decision-making model of care is a person centred approach (Rogers, 1951) in which patients, their caregivers and medical professionals work together to create a care plan and make medical decisions based on the best evidence available.

Table 6.3 Examples of communication resources for people with chronic illnesses and their caregivers.

Resource examples	Website link
Talking to others about invisible illness	**How I Talk to Others about My Invisible Illness. (2021). Carolyn Rivkees. The Daily Good Newsletter.** Access at: https://www.thegoodtrade.com/features/talking-about-invisible-illness
How to communicate with your care recipient	**Communication and Relationships. Family Caregivers Online.** Access at: https://familycaregiversonline.net/education/comm-and-relationships/
Patient education about chronic pain, illness and communication	**Patient Education Chronic Pain or Illness: Relationships and Communication. Barbara Woodward Lips. Mayo Clinic Patient Education Center.** Access at: https://texasneurology.com/assets/library/mayo-clinic-chronic-pain-or-illness-relationships-and-communication.pdf
Communication strategies to promote self-management of chronic illness	**Boxer, H. & Snyder, S. (2009). Five communication strategies to promote self-management of chronic illness. Family Practice Management, 16(5), 12-16. PMID: 19751037.** Access at: https://www.aafp.org/pubs/fpm/issues/2009/0900/p12.html

6.4.3 Managing uncertainty to improve care delivery and patient outcomes

Another area of clinical practice which should be addressed in order to improve future care is sourcing support for clinicians who are working with people with fibromyalgia-associated dysphagia. Research has found that clinicians working in this area often practise in isolation and commonly deal with uncertainty regarding the nature of these issues and their professional roles and responsibilities. Uncertainty can be moderated via the seeking of information, acknowledging and addressing unknowns, availing of non-judgemental clinical supervision, and engaging with relevant support networks and special interest

Table 6.4 Resource examples for shared decision-making conversations.

Resource examples	Website link
Fibromyalgia patient leaflet for shared decision making	**Fibromyalgia Australia: Introduction to Management, Monitoring & Communications. (2020). SA ME/CFS/FMS Clinic Research Centre / Bridges & Pathways Institute Inc.** Access at: https://fibromyalgiaaustralia.org.au/wp-content/uploads/Patient-Leaflet-05-ManagementMonitoringCommunications.pdf
Shared decision-making tool	**The SHARE Approach—Essential Steps of Shared Decision making: Expanded Reference Guide with Sample Conversation Starters. (2020). Agency for Healthcare Research and Quality, Rockville, MD.** Access at: https://www.ahrq.gov/health-literacy/professional-training/shared-decision/tool/resource-2.html
Decision-making perspectives of patients and family caregivers	**Hauser, J., Chang, C.H., Alpert, H., Baldwin, D., Emanuel, E., & Emanuel, L. (2006). Who's caring for whom? Differing perspectives between seriously ill patients and their family caregivers.** *The American Journal of Hospice & Palliative Care*, **23. 105-112. 10.1177/104990910602300207.** Access at: https://www.researchgate.net/publication/7206179_Who's_caring_for_whom_Differing_perspectives_between_seriously_ill_patients_and_their_family_caregivers
Helping patients take charge of their chronic illness	**Funnell, M.M. (2000). Helping patients take charge of their chronic illnesses.** *Family Practice Management*, **7(3), 47-51. PMID: 10947289.** Access at: https://www.aafp.org/pubs/fpm/issues/2000/0300/p47.html

research groups. Uncertainty and isolation can be mitigated via collaborative information sharing and decision making between the clinician and patient using the strategies discussed above. All of these factors can culminate to improve tolerance to uncertainty and reduce isolation, with ultimate positive impact on clinician work-related wellbeing and satisfaction and, most essentially, patient outcomes and experience (Bachman & Freeborn, 1999; Bovier & Perneger, 2007; Iannello et al., 2017).

6.5 The future of healthcare research into the experiences and management of people living with fibromyalgia-associated dysphagia

It is important for research to establish means of empathetic and holistic assessment of eating and swallowing problems among those with fibromyalgia. Patient calls for improved communication should be acknowledged in the development of standardised assessment. Furthermore, compensatory strategies reportedly most used by people living with these issues should be investigated for safety, effectiveness, and acceptability. However, while compensatory strategies are certainly an important cog in the wheel of living well with fibromyalgia-associated dysphagia, rehabilitation strategies may also be essential for people living with more severe dysphagia. Yet rehabilitation cannot begin until research establishes the true underlying physiological causes of swallowing difficulties among this group. Only when the underlying mechanism of these eating and drinking problems is known can we begin to treat them effectively from an impairment-based perspective. As such, this must be a core priority for future collaborative investigations in this field. Finally, authors here suggest that, once the above goals are achieved and a solid understanding of this condition and its effective management is gained, we draw on findings from other cohorts and promote patient-as-expert self-management educational programs into the future. As emphasised throughout this book, the patient is the true expert in living with fibromyalgia-associated dysphagia, and it is essential that their tacit wisdom and lived experience is honoured and championed through PPI activities. This collaborative model of service provision aims to empower patients and clinicians, educate them on living well with these issues, and promote positive relationships (Hoddinott et al., 2018; Luna Puerta, Bartlam, & Smith, 2019; Tembo et al., 2021;).

6.6 The first steps towards change

People with fibromyalgia-associated swallowing problems are dealing not only with the well-known multi-faceted symptom profile (e.g., pain and fatigue) but also eating and drinking problems which are often overlooked. The viewpoints of patients, caregivers, and clinicians on the current challenges to optimal care provision and symptom management have been presented here. We have also highlighted potential avenues for future collaboration and communication with the view to enhancing future care delivery and positive patient outcomes. This conversation is just beginning, and this book acts as the initial catalyst for future patient-led partnership, collaboration and communication. In this way, we can build the best practice guidelines together from a grassroots perspective to optimise care delivery and patient outcomes.

References

Abu-Snieneh, H.M. & Saleh, M.Y.N. (2018). Registered Nurses' competency to screen dysphagia among stroke patients: Literature review. *The Open Nursing Journal, 12*, 184–194. https://doi.org/10.2174/1874434601812010184

Adkins, C., Takakura, W., Spiegel, B., Lu, M., Vera-Llonch, M., Williams, J., & Almario, C. (2020). Prevalence and characteristics of dysphagia based on a population-based survey. *Clinical Gastroenterology and Hepatology: The Official Clinical Practice Journal of the American Gastroenterological Association.* https://doi.org/10.1016/j.cgh.2019.10.029

Arnold, L.M., Bennett, R.M., Crofford, L.J., Dean, L.E., Clauw, D.J., Goldenberg, D.L., & Macfarlane, G.J. (2019). AAPT diagnostic criteria for fibromyalgia. *The Journal of Pain, 20*(6), 611–628.

Arora, N.K. (2003). Interacting with cancer patients: The significance of physicians' communication behavior. *Social Science & Medicine, 57*, 791–806. http://dx.doi.org/10.1016/S0277-9536(02)00449-5

Arout, C.A., Sofuoglu, M., Bastian, L.A., & Rosenheck, R.A. (2018). Gender differences in the prevalence of fibromyalgia and in concomitant medical and psychiatric disorders: A national veterans health administration study. *Journal of Women's Health, 27*(8), 1035–1044. https://doi.org/10.1089/jwh.2017.6622

Bachman, K.H. & Freeborn, D.K. (1999). HMO physicians' use of referrals. *Social Science & Medicine, 48*(4), 547–557. https://doi.org/10.1016/s0277-9536(98)00380-3

Balasubramaniam, R., Laudenbach, J., & Stoopler, E. (2007). Fibromyalgia: An update for oral health care providers. *Oral Surgery, Oral Medicine, Oral Pathology, Oral Radiology, and Endodontology, 104*(5), 589–602. https://doi.org/10.1016/j.tripleo.2007.05.010

Belasen, A.R. & Belasen, A.T. (2018a). Dual effects of improving doctor-patient communication: Patient satisfaction and hospital ratings. Available at *SSRN 3096056*.

Belasen, A. & Belasen, A.T. (2018b). Doctor-patient communication: A review and a rationale for using an assessment framework. *Journal of Health Organization and Management, 32*(7), 891–907. https://doi.org/10.1108/JHOM-10-2017-0262

Beresford, E.B. (1991). Uncertainty and the shaping of medical decisions. *The Hastings Center Report, 21*(4), 6–11.

Bhadra, P. & Petersel, D. (2010). Medical conditions in fibromyalgia patients and their relationship to pregabalin efficacy: Pooled analysis of Phase III clinical trials. *Expert Opinion on Pharmacotherapy, 11*(17), 2805–2812. https://doi.org/10.1517/14656566.2010.525217

Bhargava, J. & Hurley, J.A. (2022). Fibromyalgia. In *StatPearls*. StatPearls Publishing. http://www.ncbi.nlm.nih.gov/books/NBK540974/

Birkeland, S., Bismark, M., Barry, M.J., & Möller, S. (2022). Is greater patient involvement associated with higher satisfaction? Experimental evidence from a vignette survey. *BMJ Quality & Safety, 31*(2), 86–93.

Bovier, P.A. & Perneger, T.V. (2007). Stress from uncertainty from graduation to retirement—a population-based study of Swiss physicians. *Journal of General Internal Medicine, 22*(5), 632–638.

Boxer, H. & Snyder, S. (2009). Five communication strategies to promote self-management of chronic illness. *Family Practice Management, 16*(5), 12–16. PMID: 19751037. Retrieved from: https://www.aafp.org/pubs/fpm/issues/2009/0900/p12.html 12/10/2022

Braun, V. & Clarke, V. (2021). *Thematic Analysis: A Practical Guide.* London: Sage.

Brédart, A., Bouleuc, C., & Dolbeault, S. (2005). Doctor-patient communication and satisfaction with care in oncology. *Current Opinion in Oncology, 17*(4), 351–354. https://doi.org/10.1097/01.cco.0000167734.26454.30

Brody, R.A., Touger-Decker, R., VonHagen, S., & Maillet, J.O. (2000). Role of registered dietitians in dysphagia screening. *Journal of the American Dietetic Association, 100*(9), 1029–1037. https://doi.org/10.1016/s0002-8223(00)00302-3

Büssing, A., Ostermann, T., Neugebauer, E.A. et al. (2010). Adaptive coping strategies in patients with chronic pain conditions and their interpretation of disease. *BMC Public Health, 10*, 507. https://doi.org/10.1186/1471-2458-10-507

Canter, J. (2021). Living well with fibromyalgia. Access at: https://www.webmd.com/fibromyalgia/guide/living-with-fibromyalgia-tips

Carroll, E., Mc Tiernan, K., & Gilheaney, Ó. (2022). An international cross-sectional survey of the current practice patterns, attitudes, and beliefs of healthcare professionals regarding eating and drinking problems in people with fibromyalgia. Poster presented at the European Society for Swallowing Disorders Conference, Leuven, Belgium, September 14–16th 2022.

Castaneda, R. (2019). Fibromyalgia self-care tips. Retrieved from: https://health.usnews.com/conditions/fibromyalgia/fibromyalgia-tips 12/10/2022

Clauw, D.J. (2014). Fibromyalgia: A clinical review. *JAMA, 311*(15), 1547–1555. https://doi.org/10.1001/jama.2014.3266

Colón León, R.A. & Centeno Vázquez, M.A. (2021). EAT-10 and Hispanics with fibromyalgia. 28th Annual Meeting of the Dysphagia Research Society. *Dysphagia, 36*, 1118–1184.

Cordier, J.F. (2014). The expert patient: Towards a novel definition. *European Respiratory Journal, 44*(4), 853–857.

Cristancho, S.M., Apramian, M.T., Vanstone, M., Lingard, L., Ott, M., & Novick, R.J. (2013). Understanding clinical uncertainty: What is going on when experienced surgeons are not sure what to do? *Academic Medicine: Journal of the Association of American Medical Colleges, 88*(10), 1516.

Davidson, E. (2021). Self-love and self-care: What chronic illness taught me about both. Retrieved from: https://creakyjoints.org/about-arthritis/rheumatoid-arthritis/ra-patient-perspectives/self-care-self-love-chronic-illness/ 12/10/2022

Davidson, E. (2022). Learning to pace myself. Retrieved from: https://creakyjoints.org/about-arthritis/rheumatoid-arthritis/ra-patient-perspectives/learning-to-pace-myself/ 14/11/2022

Davis, D.L. (2010). Simple but not always easy: Improving doctor–patient communication. *Journal of Communication in Healthcare, 3*(3–4), 240–245.

Diviney, M. & Dowling, M. (2015). Lived experiences of fibromyalgia. *Primary Health Care, 25*(9), 18–23. https//doi: 10.7748/phc.25.9.18.s27

Donaldson, L. (2003). Expert patients usher in a new era of opportunity for the NHS: The expert patient programme will improve the length and quality of lives. *Bmj, 326*(7402), 1279–1280.

Dornan, M., Semple, C., Moorhead, A., & McCaughan, E. (2021). A qualitative systematic review of the social eating and drinking experiences of patients following treatment for head and neck cancer. *Supportive Care in Cancer, 29*(9), 4899–4909.

Dorset HealthCare University NHS Foundation Trust (2022). The golden rules of swallowing (PEARS). Retrieved from: https://www.dorsethealthcare.nhs.uk/adult-speech-and-language-therapy/i-have-difficulty-swallowing-food-or-drink/golden-rules-swallowing-pears 12/07/2022

Duval, M., Black, M.A., Gesser, R., Krug, M., & Ayotte, D. (2009). Multidisciplinary evaluation and management of dysphagia: The role for otolaryngologists. *Journal of Otolaryngology–Head & Neck Surgery, 38*(2).

Ekberg, O., Hamdy, S., Woisard, V., Wuttge–Hannig, A., & Ortega, P. (2002). Social and psychological burden of dysphagia: Its impact on diagnosis and treatment. *Dysphagia, 17*(2), 139–146.

Family Caregivers Online. Communication and relationships. https://familycaregiversonline.net/education/comm-and-relationships/ 13/11/2022

Farnan, J.M., Johnson, J.K., Meltzer, D.O., Humphrey, H.J., & Arora, V.M. (2008). Resident uncertainty in clinical decision making and impact on patient care: A qualitative study. *Bmj Quality & Safety, 17*(2), 122–126.

Farneti, D. & Consolmagno, P. (2007). The Swallowing Centre: Rationale for a multidisciplinary management. *Acta Otorhinolaryngologica Italica, 27*(4), 200–207.

Farri, A., Accornero, A., & Burdese, C. (2007). Social importance of dysphagia: Its impact on diagnosis and therapy. *Acta Otorhinolaryngologica Italica, 27*(2), 83.

Fenn, M.K. & Byrne. M.(2013). The key principles of cognitive behavioral therapy. *InnovAiT, 6*(9), 579, 585.

Fibromyalgia Australia: Introduction to management, monitoring & communications. (2020). SA ME/CFS/FMS Clinic Research Centre / Bridges & Pathways Institute Inc. Retrieved from: https://fibromyalgiaaustralia.org.au/wp-content/uploads/Patient-Leaflet-05-ManagementMonitoringCommunications.pdf 13/11/2022

Fitzgerald, R.C. & Triadafilopoulos, G. (1997, February). Esophageal manifestations of rheumatic disorders. In *Seminars in Arthritis and Rheumatism, 26*(4), 641–666.

Flanagan, A. & Gilheaney, Ó. (2022). Perspectives of physicians working with patients with chronic pain dysphagia (CPD) and the challenges they face. *Dysphagia*, European Society of Swallowing Disorders Congress, Dublin, Ireland, 25–29th September 2022. https://doi.org/10.1007/s00455-022-10456-y

Fong Ha, J. & Longnecker, N. (2010). Doctor-patient communication: A review. *Ochsner Journal, 10*(1), 38–43.

Funnell, M.M. (2000). Helping patients take charge of their chronic illnesses. *Family Practice Management, 7*(3), 47–51. PMID: 10947289. https://www.aafp.org/pubs/fpm/issues/2000/0300/p47.html 13/11/2022

Galvez-Sánchez, C.M., Duschek, S., & Reyes Del Paso, G.A. (2019). Psychological impact of fibromyalgia: Current perspectives. *Psychology Research and Behavior Management, 12*, 117–127. https://doi.org/10.2147/PRBM.S178240

Garand, K.L., McCullough, G., Crary, M., Arvedson, J.C., & Dodrill, P. (2020). Assessment across the life span: The clinical swallow evaluation. *American Journal of Speech-Language Pathology, 29*(2S), 919–933. https://doi.org/10.1044/2020_AJSLP-19-00063

Gardner, B., Lally, P., & Wardle, J. (2012). Making health habitual: The psychology of 'habit-formation and general practice. *British Journal of General Practice, 62*(605), 664–666.

Gavigan, R. & Gilheaney, Ó. (2022). A qualitative investigation of the first-hand experience of dysphagia associated with fibromyalgia: An examination of online blogs. Poster presented at the European Society for Swallowing Disorders Conference, Leuven, Belgium, 14–16th September 2022.

Ghannouchi, I., Speyer, R., Doma, K., Cordier, R., & Verin, E. (2016). Swallowing function and chronic respiratory diseases: Systematic review. *Respiratory Medicine, 117*, 54–64. https://doi.org/10.1016/j.rmed.2016.05.024

Ghazanfar, H., Shehi, E., Makker, J., & Patel, H. (2021). The role of imaging modalities in diagnosing dysphagia: A clinical review. *Cureus, 13*(7).

Ghosh, A.K. (2004). Dealing with medical uncertainty: A physician's perspective. *Minnesota Medicine, 87*(10), 48–51.

Gilheaney, Ó. & Chadwick, A. (2023). The prevalence and nature of eating and swallowing problems in adults with fibromyalgia: A systematic review. *Dysphagia*, 1–17.

Gilheaney, Ó. & McTiernan, K. (2023, May). The FibroForum Conference Website. https://fibroforumtcd.online/

Gilheaney, Ó., Costello, C., & Mc Tiernan, K. [In Press] Surveying the international prevalence and nature of eating, drinking and swallowing difficulties in adults presenting with Fibromyalgia. *Dysphagia*.

Godwin, E. & Rogers, K. (2016). Integrated physiotherapy and speech pathology dysphagia assessment and treatment: A single pediatric case study. *Perspectives of the ASHA Special Interest Groups, 1*(13), 17–25. https://doi.org/10.1044/persp1.SIG13.17

Grant, P.D., Morgan, D.E., Scholz, F.J., & Canon, C.L. (2009). Pharyngeal dysphagia: What the radiologist needs to know. *Current Problems in Diagnostic Radiology, 38*(1), 17–32. https://doi.org/10.1067/j.cpradiol.2007.08.009

Grilo, A.M., Santos, M.C.d., Isabel Gomes, A., & Rita, J.S. (2017). Promoting patient-centered care in chronic disease. In *Patient Centered Medicine*. IntechOpen. https://doi.org/10.5772/67380

Gulbrandsen, P. (2020). Shared decision making: Improving doctor-patient communication. *BMJ, 368*, doi: https://doi.org/10.1136/bmj.m97

Funnell, M.M. (2000). Helping patients take charge of their chronic illnesses. *Family Practice Management, 7*(3), 47–51. PMID: 10947289. Retrieved from: https://www.aafp.org/pubs/fpm/issues/2000/0300/p47.html 13/11/2022

Hauser, J., Chang, C.H., Alpert, H., Baldwin, D., Emanuel, E., & Emanuel, L. (2006). Who's caring for whom? Differing perspectives between seriously ill patients and their family caregivers. *The American Journal of Hospice & Palliative Care, 23*, 105–112. https://doi.org/10.1177/104990910602300207

Häuser, W., Ablin, J., Fitzcharles, M.-A., Littlejohn, G., Luciano, J.V., Usui, C., & Walitt, B. (2015). Fibromyalgia. *Nature Reviews. Disease Primers, 1*, 15022. https://doi.org/10.1038/nrdp.2015.22

Hawken, T., Turner-Cobb, J., & Barnett, J. (2018). Coping and adjustment in caregivers: A systematic review. *Health Psychology Open, 5*(2), 2055102918810659

Helou, M.A., DiazGranados, D., Ryan, M.S., & Cyrus, J.W. (2020). Uncertainty in decision-making in medicine: A scoping review and thematic analysis of conceptual models. *Academic Medicine: Journal of the Association of American Medical Colleges, 95*(1), 157–165. https://doi.org/10.1097/ACM.0000000000002902

Herndon, J.H. & Pollick, K. (2002). Continuing concerns, new challenges, and next steps in physician-patient communication. *JBJS, 84*(2), 309–315.

Hillen, M.A., Gutheil, C.M., Strout, T.D., Smets, E.M., & Han, P.K. (2017). Tolerance of uncertainty: Conceptual analysis, integrative model, and implications for healthcare. *Social Science & Medicine, 180*, 62–75.

Hobma, S., Ram, P., Muijtjens, A., Vleuten, C. van der, & Grol, R. (2006). Effective improvement of doctor–patient communication: A randomised controlled trial. *British Journal of General Practice, 56*(529), 580–586.

Hoddinott, P., Pollock, A., O'Cathain, A., Boyer, I., Taylor, J., MacDonald, C., Oliver, S., & Donovan, J.L. (2018). How to incorporate patient and public perspectives into the design and conduct of research. *F1000Research, 7*, 752. https://doi.org/10.12688/f1000research.15162.1

Hollenbach, M., Feisthammel, J., Mössner, J., & Hoffmeister, A. (2018). Dysphagia from a gastroenterologist's perspective. *Deutsche Medizinische Wochenschrift, 143*(9), 660–671. https://doi.org/10.1055/s-0043-113713

Hughes, T.a.T. & Wiles, C.M. (1998). Neurogenic dysphagia: The role of the neurologist. *Journal of Neurology, Neurosurgery & Psychiatry, 64*(5), 569–572. https://doi.org/10.1136/jnnp.64.5.569

Hussey, J. & Gilheaney, Ó. (2022). The effect of eating, drinking, and swallowing difficulties on people with fibromyalgia: A qualitative analysis of personal experiences. Presented at the 12th European Society for Swallowing Disorders, Leuven, Belgium, 12–16th September 2022.

Iannello, P., Mottini, A., Tirelli, S., Riva, S., & Antonietti, A. (2017). Ambiguity and uncertainty tolerance, need for cognition, and their association with stress. A study among Italian practicing physicians. *Medical Education Online, 22*(1), 1270009.

Irfan, B., Irfan, O., Ansari, A. Qidwai, W., & Nanji, K. (2017). Impact of caregiving on various aspects of the lives of caregivers. *Cureus, 9*(5), e1213. doi: 10.7759/cureus.1213. PMID: 28589062; PMCID: PMC5453737

Jalilvand, A.D., Belle, P., McNally, M., & Perry, K.A. (2019). Functional gastrointestinal and neurologic disorders may alter gastroesophageal reflux disease presentation and post-operative symptomology and quality of life following Nissen Fundoplication. *Gastroenterology, 156,*(6), S1463–S1463.

Jeon, Y. (2020). Fibromyalgia: Practical considerations for oral health care providers. *Journal of Dental Anesthesia and Pain Medicine, 20*(5), 263.

Kennedy, A., Rogers, A., & Bower, P. (2007). Support for self-care for patients with chronic disease. *Bmj,10*, 335(7627), 968–970. doi: 10.1136/bmj.39372.540903.94. PMID: 17991978; PMCID: PMC2071971

Kim, G.M., Lim, J.Y., Kim, E.J., & Park, S.M. (2019). Resilience of patients with chronic diseases: A systematic review. *Health & Social Care in the Community, 4*, 797–807. doi: 10.1111/hsc.12620. Epub 2018 Jul 20. PMID: 30027595

Kim, K. & Lee, Y.-M. (2018). Understanding uncertainty in medicine: Concepts and implications in medical education. *Korean Journal of Medical Education, 30*(3), 181–188. https://doi.org/10.3946/kjme.2018.92

Kindler, C., Szirt, L., Sommer, D., Haeusler, R., & Langewitz, W. (2005). A quantitative analysis of anaesthetist-patient communication during the pre-operative visit. *Anaesthesia, 60*, 53–59. 10.1111/j.1365-2044.2004.03995.x

Korzh, O. & Tsodikova, O. (2019). Improving doctor-patient communication in a primary care setting. *Romanian Journal of Medical Practice, 14*, 12–16.

Kurtz, S.M. (2002). Doctor-patient communication: Principles and practices. *Canadian Journal of Neurological Sciences, 29*(S2), S23–S29.

Lancaster, J. (2015). Dysphagia: Its nature, assessment and management. *British Journal of Community Nursing (Suppl Nutrition)*, S28–S32. https://doi.org/10.12968/bjcn.2015.20. Sup6a.S28

Lillie, S.F., Haines, J., Vyas, A., & Fowler, S.J. (2014). P121 Speech And Language Therapy in pulmonary rehabilitation: The implication of education sessions on dysphagia management. *Thorax, 69* (Suppl 2), A131–A131. https://doi.org/10.1136/thoraxjnl-2014-206260.262

Lisiecka, D., Kelly, H., & Jackson, J. (2021). How do people with Motor Neurone Disease experience dysphagia? A qualitative investigation of personal experiences. *Disability and Rehabilitation, 43*(4), 479–488.

Logemann, J.A. (1994). Multidisciplinary management of dysphagia. *Acta Oto-Rhino-Laryngologica Belgica, 48*(2), 235–238.

Luca, N.R., Smith, M., & Hibbert, S. (2022). A community-based participatory research approach to understanding social eating for food well-being. *Emerald Open Research, 3*, 11.

Luna Puerta, L., Bartlam, B., & Smith, H.E. (2019). Researchers' perspectives on public involvement in health research in Singapore: The argument for a community-based approach. *Health Expectations, 22*(4), 666–675.

Lundquist, M.C. (2019). A guide to caregiver self-care. Retrieved from: https://www. care2caregivers.com/wp-content/uploads/2019/12/Caregiver-Self-Care-Booklet-English. pdf 13/11/2022

Macleod, M. & O'Shea, S. (2019). The dietitian's role in diagnosis and treatment of dysphagia. In O. Ekberg (Ed.), *Dysphagia: Diagnosis and Treatment*, pp.717–729. Springer International Publishing. https://doi.org/10.1007/174_2017_124

MacNamara, M. (2022). Dysphagia and communication difficulties associated with fibromyalgia: A qualitative exploration of family members', carers' and loved ones' experiences. Unpublished Undergraduate Thesis. Trinity College Dublin.

Marín-Maicas, P., Corchón, S., Ambrosio, L., & Portillo, M.C. (2021). Living with long term conditions from the perspective of family caregivers. A scoping review and narrative synthesis. *International Journal of Environmental Research & Public Health, 18*(14), 72–94. doi: 10.3390/ijerph18147294. PMID: 34299745; PMCID: PMC8305191

Martire, L.M. & Helgeson, V.S. (2017). Close relationships and the management of chronic illness: Associations and interventions. *American Psychology, 72*(6), 601–612. doi: 10.1037/amp0000066. PMID: 28880106; PMCID: PMC5598776

Mayo Clinic Staff. (2022). Caregiver stress: Tips for taking care of yourself. https://www. mayoclinic.org/healthy-lifestyle/stress-management/in-depth/caregiver-stress/art-20044784 18/11/2022

McCabe, R. & Healey, P.G. (2018). Miscommunication in doctor–patient communication. *Topics in Cognitive Science, 10*(2), 409–424.

McKinstry, A., Tranter, M., & Sweeney, J. (2010). Outcomes of dysphagia intervention in a pulmonary rehabilitation program. *Dysphagia, 25*(2), 104–111. https://doi.org/10.1007/s00455-009-9230-3

Megari, K. (2013). Quality of life in chronic disease patients. *Health Psychology Research, 1*(3), e27. doi: 10.4081/hpr.2013.e27. PMID: 26973912; PMCID: PMC4768563

Meryn, S. (1998). Improving doctor-patient communication. *Bmj, 316*(7149), 1922–1930.

NHS. (2022). Diagnosis – dysphagia (swallowing problems). Retrieved from: https://www. nhs.uk/conditions/swallowing-problems-dysphagia/diagnosis/ 11/07/2022

National Health Service. (2022). Overview – dysphagia (swallowing problems). Retrieved from: Dysphagia (swallowihttps://www.nhs.uk/conditions/swallowing-problems-dysphagia/ng problems) - NHS (www.nhs.uk) 21/11/2022

Neeman, N., Isaac, T., Leveille, S., Dimonda, C., Shin, J.Y., Aronson, M.D., & Freedman, S.D. (2012). Improving doctor–patient communication in the outpatient setting using a facilitation tool: A preliminary study. *International Journal for Quality in Health Care, 24*(4), 357–364. https://doi.org/10.1093/intqhc/mzr081

Ninfa, A., Crispiatico, V., Pizzorni, N., Bassi, M., Casazza, G., Schindler, A., & Delle Fave, A. (2021). The care needs of persons with oropharyngeal dysphagia and their informal caregivers: A scoping review. *PloS one, 16*(9), e0257683.

Nutricia (2022). Your guide to safe swallowing and easy eating - Information booklet for patients and carers. Retrieved from: https://www.nutricia.ie/content/dam/dam/amn/local/gb/approved/nutricia/guide-to-safe-swallowing-and-easy-eating.pdf 05/07/2022

Ogden, J. (2019). *Health Psychology*. London: McGraw-Hill.

Piersala, K., Akst, L.M., Hillel, A.T., & Best, S.R. (2020). Chronic pain syndromes and their laryngeal manifestations. *JAMA Otolaryngology – Head & Neck Surgery, 146*(6), 543–549. https://doi.org/10.1001/jamaoto.2020.0530

Pizzorni, N. (2017). Social and psychologic impact of dysphagia. In O. Ekberg (Ed.) *Dysphagia. Medical Radiology*. Springer, Cham. https://doi.org/10.1007/174_2017_132

Reinstein, A. (2020). Diagnosing dysphagia: What are we looking for? Retrieved from: https://www.amyspeechlanguagetherapy.com/guidelines-for-safe-swallowing.html 12/07/2022

Remson, S. (2022). Have you been budgeting your spoons this school year? Retrieved from: https://creakyjoints.org/about-arthritis/rheumatoid-arthritis/ra-patient-perspectives/budgeting-spoons-this-school-year/ 14/11/2022

Rhodus, N.L., Fricton, J., Carlson, P., & Messner, R. (2003). Oral symptoms associated with fibromyalgia syndrome. *The Journal of Rheumatology, 30*(8), 1841–1845.

Richards, T. (1990). Chasms in communication. *Bmj, 301*(6766), 1407.

Rivkees, C. (2021). How I talk to others about my invisible illness. *The Daily Good Newsletter*. Retrieved from: https://www.thegoodtrade.com/features/talking-about-invisible-illness 13/11/2022

Rogers, C. (1951). *Client-centered Therapy: Its Current Practice, Implications and Theory*. London: Constable.

Rouleau, G., Bélisle-Pipon, J.C., Birko, S., Karazivan, P., Fernandez, N., Bilodeau, K., & Rodrigue, C. (2018). Early career researchers' perspectives and roles in patient-oriented research. *Research Involvement and Engagement, 4*(1), 1–15.

Rowe, R.A., Fuschia M., Sirois, F.M., Toussaint, L., Kohls, N., Nöfer, E., Offenbächer, M., Jameson, K., & Hirsch, J.K. (2019). Health beliefs, attitudes, and health-related quality of life in persons with fibromyalgia: Mediating role of treatment adherence. *Psychology, Health & Medicine, 24*(8), 962–977. doi: 10.1080/13548506.2019.1576913

Sarzi-Puttini, P., Atzeni, F., Clauw, D.J., & Perrot, S. (2015). The impact of pain on systemic rheumatic diseases. *Best Practice & Research Clinical Rheumatology, 29*(1), 1–5.

Sarzi-Puttini, P., Giorgi, V., Marotto, D., & Atzeni, F. (2020). Fibromyalgia: An update on clinical characteristics, aetiopathogenesis and treatment. *Nature Reviews. Rheumatology, 16*(11), 645–660. https://doi.org/10.1038/s41584-020-00506-w

Sasegbon, A. & Hamdy, S. (2017). The anatomy and physiology of normal and abnormal swallowing in oropharyngeal dysphagia. *Neurogastroenterology & Motility, 29*(11), e13100.

Schultz, K. (2019). I'm a "Spoonie." Here's what I wish more people knew about chronic illness. Access at: https://www.healthline.com/health/spoon-theory-chronic-illness-explained-like-never-before#1

Seccia, T.M., Rossitto, G., Calò, L.A., & Rossi, G.P. (2015). Oral burning with dysphagia and weight loss. *Medicine, 94*(31), e1163. doi/10.1097/MD.0000000000001163

Sherman, D.W., Austin A., Jones, S., Stimmerman, T., & Tamayo, M. (2016). Shifting attention to the family caregiver: The neglected, vulnerable, at-risk person sitting at the side of your patient and struggling to maintain their own health. *Journal of Family Medicine, 3*(7), 1080. https://austinpublishinggroup.com/family-medicine/fulltext/jfm-v3-id1080.pdf

Smith, E., Bélisle-Pipon, J.C., & Resnik, D. (2019). Patients as research partners: How to value their perceptions, contribution and labor? *Citizen Science, 4*(1), 10.5334/cstp.184. doi: 10.5334/cstp.184. PMID: 32064121; PMCID: PMC7021275

Stewart, M.A. (1995). Effective physician-patient communication and health outcomes: A review. *CMAJ: CanadianMedical Association Journal, 152*(9), 1423.

Stojanovic, M., Fries, S., & Grund, A. (2021). Self-efficacy in habit building: How general and habit-specific self-efficacy influence behavioral automatization and motivational interference. *Frontiers of Psychology,12*, 643753. doi: 10.3389/fpsyg.2021.643753. PMID: 34025512; PMCID: PMC8137900

Stone, M. (2014). Prescribing in patients with dysphagia. *Nurse Prescribing, 12*(10). https://doi.org/10.12968/npre.2014.12.10.504

Stoewen, D.L. (2017). Dimensions of wellness: Change your habits, change your life. *Canadian Veterinary Journal, 58*(8), 861–862. PMID: 28761196; PMCID: PMC5508938

Sullivan, A.B. & Miller D. (2015). Who is taking care of the caregiver? *Journal of Patient Experience, 2*(1), 7-12. doi:10.1177/237437431500200103

Tembo, D., Hickey, G., Montenegro, C., Chandler, D., Nelson, E., Porter, K., ... & Rennard, U. (2021). Effective engagement and involvement with community stakeholders in the co-production of global health research. *Bmj, 372*, n178.

The Agency for Healthcare Research and Quality. (2020). The SHARE Approach—Essential steps of shared decision making: Expanded reference guide with sample conversation starters. The Agency for Healthcare Research and Quality, Rockville, MD. Retrieved from: https://www.ahrq.gov/health-literacy/professional-training/shared-decision/tool/resource-2.html 12/09/2022

The American Association of Occupational Therapists (2011). Occupational Therapy: A vital role in dysphagia care: Fact sheet. Retrieved from: https://www.aota.org/~/media/Corporate/Files/AboutOT/Professionals/WhatIsOT/RDP/Facts/Dysphagia%20fact%20sheet.pdf 12/07/2022

The American Speech-Language-Hearing Association (2022). Adult dysphagia. Retrieved from: https://www.asha.org/practice-portal/clinical-topics/adult-dysphagia/#collapse_4 12/07/2022

The Family Caregiver Alliance. (2022). Taking care of YOU: Self-care for family caregivers. Retrieved from: https://www.caregiver.org/resource/taking-care-you-self-care-family-caregivers/ 11/10/2022

The Regents of the University of California. (2022). Self-care for caregivers. Retrieved from: https://www.ucsfhealth.org/education/self-care-for-caregivers 10/11/2022

Tomik, J., Sowula, K., Ceranowicz, P., Dworak, M., & Stolcman, K. (2020). Effects of biofeedback training on esophageal peristalsis in amyotrophic lateral sclerosis patients with dysphagia. *Journal of Clinical Medicine*, *9*(7), 2314. https://dx.doi.org/10.3390/JCM9072314

Tongue, J.R., Epps, H.R., & Forese, L.L. (2005). Communication skills for patient-centered care: Research-based, easily learned techniques for medical interviews that benefit orthopaedic surgeons and their patients. *JBJS*, *87*(3), 652–658.

Tracey, I. & Bushnell, M.C. (2009). How neuroimaging studies have challenged us to rethink: Is chronic pain a disease? *The Journal of Pain*, *10*(11), 1113–1120.

Vivino, F.B., Bunya, V.Y., Massaro-Giordano, G., Johr, C.R., Giattino, S.L., Schorpion, A., ... & Ambrus Jr, J.L. (2019). Sjogren's syndrome: An update on disease pathogenesis, clinical manifestations and treatment. *Clinical Immunology (Orlando, Fla.)*, *203*, 81–121.

Wei, M. (2018). Self-care for the caregiver. Retrieved from: https://www.health.harvard.edu/blog/self-care-for-the-caregiver-2018101715003 14/11/2022

White, K., Issac, M.S., Kamoun, C., Leygues, J., & Cohn, S. (2018). The THRIVE model: A framework and review of internal and external predictors of coping with chronic illness. *Health Psychology Open*, *5*(2), 2055102918793552. doi: 10.1177/2055102918793552. PMID: 30151224; PMCID: PMC6104221

Woolf, C.J. (2011). Central sensitization: Implications for the diagnosis and treatment of pain. *Pain*, *152*(3), S2–S15.

Wolfe, F., Clauw, D.J., Fitzcharles, M.A., Goldenberg, D.L., Katz, R.S., Mease, P., Russell, A.S., Russell, I.J., Winfield, J.B., & Yunus, M.B. (2010). The American College of Rheumatology preliminary diagnostic criteria for fibromyalgia and measurement of symptom severity. *Arthritis Care & Research*, *62*(5), 600–610. https://doi.org/10.1002/acr.20140

Woodward Lips, B. (2022). Patient education chronic pain or illness: Relationships and communication. Mayo Clinic Patient Education Center. Retrieved from: https://texasneurology.com/assets/library/mayo-clinic-chronic-pain-or-illness-relationships-and-communication.pdf 14/11/2022

Wright, D., Begent, D., & Crawford, H. (2017). Concensus Guideline on the medication management of adults with swallowing difficulties. Mebendium Group, Buckinghamshire, UK.

Index